'In this important and timely exploration of the nature of knowledge, Brothers and Sletvold address the heart of the therapeutic endeavor and the question of what it means to be human. They demonstrate unequivocally that knowing and understanding are never individual achievements, but fundamentally relational and embodied in nature, shaped by historical circumstances and our interactions with others. They invite us to learn from and live with uncertainty and thus to recognize that experience may be more or less known, formulated or unformulated, in any moment in time.'

Roger Frie, *Professor of Psychoanalysis and Education, University of Vienna, Austria*

'*Psychoanalytic Explorations of Embodied Relational Knowing* is a unique, and fascinating work, which probes the nature of knowledge in clinical and cultural contexts. Drawing on philosophy and psychoanalytic theory, the authors explore the way that traumatic knowledge is inscribed on the body. The body's truths are in perpetual tension with the human desire to not know. This tension—between knowing and not-knowing—is present in clinical process, and it has diverse meanings. It is also fundamental to the authoritarian turn that we see throughout the globe. In its examination, this book spans the personal, the historical and the political.'

Sue Grand, *PhD, Author,* The Reproduction of Evil: A Clinical and Cultural Perspective

'Doris Brothers and Jon Sletvold's title *Psychoanalytic Explorations of Embodied Relational Knowing* concentrates in three words a wealth of clinical experience concerning the limits of psychoanalysis. It is when we are confronted with the inadequacy of speech and experience—the total loneliness at the outer edges of relationships—that the impasse created by the conflict between "the need to know and to be known" and "not to know and not to be known" is overcome by "embodied relational knowing." The authors are supported by philosophers and authors whom Freud claims, in the "Gradiva," to be his "precious allies." By drawing on examples from their clinical practices, they provide a source of great learning and hope for their readers.'

Françoise Davoine, *PhD, Author,* Wittgenstein's Folly

'Doris Brothers' and Jon Sletvold's exploration of "embodied relational knowing" does well to advance our understanding of what transpires not only in the context of therapeutic dialogue but in our ongoing engagement with the world. For Brothers and Sletvold, the world is inscribed within us; it is embedded and embodied, in ways both known and unknown. There can thus be no illusions of fully containing who and what we—and others—are. That's not what we seek in any case. For the desire to know and be known cannot ever be teased apart from the desire not to know and not to be known. Whether what's being explored is traumatic dissociation or madness or silence in the face of patent evil, this thoughtful, wise, humane book shows that the need to know and not know is carried forth pervasively and, often, surreptitiously, in the very flesh of our being and the very fabric of our relationships.'

Mark Freeman, *PhD, Distinguished Professor of Ethics and Society Emeritus, College of the Holy Cross, and Senior Fellow, Center for Psychological Humanities and Ethics, Boston College, author of* Toward the Psychological Humanities: A Modest Manifesto for the Future of Psychology

'This is a book about the human need to know—and not to know. Brothers and Sletvold look to the body to better understand our instinct to seek knowledge about ourselves and our world, foregrounding how emotion, perception and sensory-motor processes go into what we can know about our patients and their situations. This is a sophisticated boundary-pushing book set forth in unpretentious, conversational prose.'

Daniel Goldin, *PsyD, Editor,* Psychoanalytic Inquiry

Psychoanalytic Explorations of Embodied Relational Knowing

This book offers groundbreaking insights into relational theory, exploring the patient's and the analyst's longings to know, be known and not known in psychoanalytic relationships, and the embodied nature of the healing process.

Recognition of the patient's unknowable uniqueness, which is not fully accessible by means of empathy, is shown to promote more ethical therapeutic practices. Although few psychoanalytic books have highlighted the work of the philosopher, Marcel Foucault, Brothers and Sletvold find much that is highly relevant in his work. They also demonstrate the powerful influence of culture, history, politics and world events on the therapeutic encounter.

With an informed and compassionate perspective, this book is essential reading for psychoanalysts and psychotherapists regardless of their theoretical orientation.

Doris Brothers is a co-founder of the Training and Research in Intersubjective Self Psychology Foundation. She was a co-editor of *Psychoanalysis, Self and Context* with Roger Frie from 2015 to 2019 and is consulting editor of *Psychoanalytic Inquiry*. She has written four books including *Toward a Psychology of Uncertainty Trauma-Centered Psychoanalysis* (2008) and many journal articles. She practices on the upper west side of Manhattan, New York, USA, and in Oslo, Norway.

Jon Sletvold is the founding board director of the Norwegian Character Analytic Institute. He has published books and articles on the role of the body in psychoanalysis and psychotherapy. He is the author of *The Embodied Analyst: From Freud and Reich to Relationality* (2014), winner of the Gradiva Award in 2015. He is co-director with Doris Brothers of the Wilhelm Reich Center for the Study of Embodiment.

Psychoanalytic Explorations of Embodied Relational Knowing

Doris Brothers and Jon Sletvold

Routledge
Taylor & Francis Group
LONDON AND NEW YORK

Designed cover image: © Fred De Noyelle/GODONG/Getty Images

First published 2027
by Routledge
4 Park Square, Milton Park, Abingdon, Oxon OX14 4RN

and by Routledge
605 Third Avenue, New York, NY 10158

Routledge is an imprint of the Taylor & Francis Group, an informa business

British Library Cataloguing-in-Publication Data
A catalogue record for this book is available from the British Library

ISBN: 9781032784403 (hbk)
ISBN: 9781032784380 (pbk)
ISBN: 9781003487883 (ebk)

DOI: 10.4324/9781003487883

Typeset in Optima
by Newgen Publishing UK

Contents

Acknowledgments

Even before we wrote the first pages of this book we hoped that our friends and colleagues would welcome it. What we couldn't have known in advance was the generous help so many of them have given us.

We feel especially grateful to the members of our supervision/study group for the thoughtful way they dialogued with us about the contents of each chapter and bravely experimented with our new approach to embodied supervision. Our heartfelt thanks go to Heather Demeter, Gabrielle Ducsay, Diane Fremont, Greta Laine, Teodor Negulescu, Ramona Popescu, Vincent Stephen, Alexandra Tenebroso, Georges Tremblay and Tomas.

We are deeply moved by the extraordinary contributions to our chapter on the world that we received from Stacy Berlin, Mark Freeman, Sue Grand, Daniel Goldin, Lynne Jacobs, Thato Letsatsi, Maxwell Sucharov, Ilene Philipsen and Haim Weinberg. We are also indebted to Louis Sass for allowing us to use excerpts from his forthcoming book on envy.

The love and support we received from our children, grandchildren and our dear friends in New York and Oslo has nourished us throughout this writing project.

It is difficult to express the depth of the gratitude we feel for our patients. By teaching us about their needs to know and be known as well as their needs not to know and not to be known, they have helped us to understand ourselves more deeply and hopefully to become better at healing.

We thank Kate Hawes, Senior Publisher for Global Mental Health, Routledge for her unfailing support, Aakriti Aggarwal and MaryKathryn Underwood editorial assistants, for their wise counsel, and Clarrisa Ryan for her beautiful cover illustration.

Introduction to Embodied Relational Knowing

It might be said that we analysts are in the business of knowing. Most of us work hard at knowing all that we can about ourselves and our patients. But how well we know depends, to some extent, on what we have learned. We need to have learned which theories best guide our work and how they might apply to each patient's particular concerns. We need to have learned something of history, culture, science, the arts and world events to enrich and complexify our therapeutic encounters. We need to have learned how to attend to our bodily reactions and to those of our patients if we are to understand the vast array of emotional experiences that cannot be expressed verbally. But perhaps most importantly, we need to learn the limits of what we can know about ourselves and our patients. We also need to learn how to reach beyond these limits.

Our concept of embodied relational knowing is based on the idea that limitations in our ability to know ourselves and others often give rise to needs (sometimes experienced as longings) to be known by others—known for all our weaknesses and strengths, our pains and our pleasures, our shameful failings and our proud accomplishments—and to know others as deeply and completely. The impossibility of the complete fulfillment of these needs does not preclude our strivings.

Embodied relational knowing also includes our needs not to be known and not to know others. While these needs become apparent within the context of traumatic dissociation, we view them as pervasive aspects of everyday life.

There are times when the needs to know and be known seem to intertwine with the needs not to know or not to be known. This happens in various ways. For example, we may not be able to integrate what our bodies know—what is nonverbal and implicit—with our conscious cognitive knowing. This experiential discrepancy, we believe, is involved in many challenging therapeutic encounters. It figures importantly in considering what is available to consciousness and what is not in situations involving traumatic dissociation. We believe that it is likely to be particularly marked in certain experiences of madness and when hatred develops between analysts and patients. We call attention to the curious linking of knowing and not knowing in our discussion

DOI: 10.4324/9781003487883-1

of dreams and their simultaneous collision at times of societal upheaval in a chapter on knowing the world.

We want to make it clear that we are not endorsing a Cartesian split between mind and body and a valuing of the thinking mind over feelings and bodily sensations. Rather, for us, cognitive knowing is as completely and inescapably embodied as what is experienced on a bodily level. Moreover, nothing that is known in either realm is infallible.

We are greatly indebted to Roger Frie (2017) for conceptualizing the intertwining of knowing and not knowing with respect to his discovery that his beloved grandfather had been a member of the NSKK or National Socialist Motor Corps, a paramilitary organization of the Nazi party in Germany during World War II. We are in full agreement with the following statement by Frie:

> Following Sullivan, I find it useful to think of human understanding in terms of a continuum of possibilities for knowing and not knowing. These possibilities are generated in our relationships with other people and the contexts in which we live. It is through the exploration of our relational worlds that we may come to appreciate the nature of remembering and forgetting. Experience may be more or less known, formulated or unformulated, and any moment in time, depending on the social interactions and historical circumstances in which we find ourselves.
>
> (Frie, 2017, p. 178)

We have found that the needs that comprise relational knowing, which are often intensified in the context of faulty relationships as well as by traumas, organize much that transpires in therapeutic relationships. While these needs are not often verbally expressed or even consciously experienced, they may strongly motivate people to enter therapeutic relationships. Many hope to find in their therapist, someone who will finally fulfill all their unmet needs for relational knowing. With the increased fulfillment of these needs, more of what was previously known only on a bodily level may come to be known cognitively. This tends to improve experiences of embodied wholeness and wellbeing.

We have come to believe that much that occurs between patients and therapists involves traumatic experiences in their own lives, in their parents and grandparents' lives, as well as in the world around them (see Brothers & Sletvold, 2023a, 2023b, 2023c). We contend that however it occurs, trauma confronts us with the uncertainty of what Winnicott (1965) termed "going-on-being," We have the idea that our intense interest in knowing about ourselves, others, our planet and our universe reflects not only the obvious fact that we humans are curious beings, but that we often feel that our very survival depends on what we know—and what we don't want to know. If, as we have suggested, we inhabit a world suffused with trauma and trauma confronts us with the unbearable sense of uncertainty about our going on being, knowing—however incomplete, provides us with some illusion of certainty. At the same time, to the extent that our needs not to know or be known serve to simplify experience, they may also reduce experiences of uncertainty.

We have suggested that the aim of psychoanalytic therapy is not to heal trauma per se; the very efforts undertaken to restore certainty in the aftermath of traumatic experiences often lead to relational difficulties that require therapeutic attention. Many of the clinical examples that we provide in this book reflect the ways in which our relational knowing needs that are intensified in the hope of reducing a sense of uncertainty, organize therapeutic relationships. We also demonstrate ways of working with patients that make use of their embodied sense of knowing themselves and others.

Philosophical Underpinnings

The concept of knowing is often related to the branch of philosophy known as epistemology. Our understanding of ourselves and the world has been greatly influenced by such well-known epistemologists as Plato, Aristotle, Descartes, Spinoza and Leibniz. Beginning with Freud, many philosophers and psychoanalysts have examined the ways in which various philosophical perspectives underpin knowledge in psychoanalysis. Most of these perspectives support our understanding that our knowledge of ourselves and others is never complete.

Stänicke, Zachrisson & Vetleseen (2020), for example, suggest that Freud was influenced by Kant's transcendental idealism. As they point out, Freud portrays humans as lacking a direct view of reality. Consider how Freud references Kant in his 1915 paper, "the Unconscious":

> Just as Kant warned us not to overlook the fact that our perceptions are subjectively conditioned and must not be regarded as identical with what is perceived though unknowable, so psychoanalysis warns us not to equate perceptions by means of consciousness with the unconscious mental processes which are their object.
>
> (1915, p. 171)

When Freud later developed the concept of primary and secondary process thinking and the pleasure and the reality principles, he concluded that the way we perceive the world is never undisturbed; it is always influenced by wishes, hopes and fears. To the end of his life, Freud maintained that our relation to reality is uncertain, and he advised analysts to be modest about their truth claims.

The philosophical perspectives applied to psychoanalysis following Freud, run the gamut. Habermas (1972) and Ricoeur (1970), for example, argue that psychoanalysis should be regarded as a hermeneutical endeavor. Others suggest a constructivist perspective. In his 1999 book, *The Creation of Reality in Psychoanalysis*, Richard Moore examines the philosophical perspectives of Donald Spence and Roy Schafer on narrative truth, Robert Stolorow's views on intersubjectivity theory and Irwin Hoffman's constructivist perspective. He criticizes these theorists for failing to develop a thorough-going constructivist understanding without retreating to what he considers "the safe haven of positivism," which, for Moore, involves any understanding that goes beyond subjective experience.

As Donna Orange (2003) points out in a review of Richard Moore's book, intersubjective-systems theory, which she developed with Robert Stolorow and George Atwood, is best understood as a phenomenological contextualism insofar as it investigates emotional experience that takes form in constitutive intersubjective contexts.

We also locate the source of our ideas within the philosophical framework known as phenomenology, particularly as it is explicated by Maurice Merleau-Ponty. We have drawn on Merleau-Ponty's (1962) understanding that "we find in ourselves, and nowhere else, the true meaning of phenomenology" (p. viii).

He explains:

> All my knowledge of the world, even my scientific knowledge, is gained from my own particular point of view, or from some experience of the world without which the symbols of science would be meaningless.
>
> (Merleau-Ponty, 1962, p. viii)

Our ideas build on Merleau-Ponty's assertion that we "know all things from a particular perspective" which, he notes, "is informed by "my education, my previous efforts, my personal history" (1962, p.61).

Merleau-Ponty's formulations are highly congruent with Nietzche's (1887/2017) concept of perspectivism. Consider the following:

> Let us be on guard against the dangerous old conceptual fiction that posited a "pure, will-less, painless, timeless knowing subject:" let us guard against the snare of contradictory concepts as "pure reason," "absolute spirituality," "knowledge in itself": these always demand that we should think of an eye that is completely unthinkable, an eye turned in no direction, in which the active and interpreting forces, though which seeing becomes seeing *something*, are supposed to be lacking; these always demand of the eye an absurdity and a nonsense. There is *only* perspective seeing, *only* perspective knowing, and the *more* affects we allow to speak about one thing, the *more* eyes, different eyes, we can use to observe one thing, the more complete will our "concept" of this thing, our "objectivity" be.
>
> (Nietzche, 1887/2017, p. 12)

Allison Merrick (2025), refers to Nietsche in describing what she calls "the nature of knowers." She observes:

> Knowers, for Nietzsche, are embedded in historical, socio-political systems, and embodied with interests, desires, and affects. When we encounter knowers, then, we find them not as disembodied intellects but as beings situated within social, historical, and political contexts that shape as they constrain their modes of understanding. Knowers are, further still, animated by interests, permeated by desire, and enmeshed in conflicts that shape what they want to know and what they come to know. This is what it means for a knower to have a perspective . . . a perspective is an essential prerequisite of knowing.
>
> (Merrick, 2025)

To the extent that embodied relational knowing is constituted by needs, we believe it aligns both with Nietzche's understanding of knowers and falls within the realm that Merleau-Ponty describes as phenomenological. The needs to know and be known as well as the needs not to know or be known arise from each person's unique encounters with others and are shaped by one's social, cultural and historical heritage. They are formed within the world one inhabits and the worlds of one's ancestors. We are in full agreement with Merleau-Ponty's (1962) assertion:

> Truth does not inhabit only the inner man, or more accurately, there is no inner man, man is in the world, and only in the world does he know himself.
>
> (Merleau-Ponty, 1962, p. xi)

Our work is also indebted to Merleau-Ponty's emphasis on embodiment insofar as we understand relational knowing to develop among what we term, "talking bodies." It is not only by means of language that we know ourselves and others but in the myriad nonverbal forms of communication that link us to one another. The following quote aptly captures his understanding:

> My body is the fabric into which all objects are woven, the general instrument of my "comprehension." It is my body which gives significance not only to the natural object but also to cultural objects like words.
>
> (Merleau-Ponty, 1962, p.235)

Merleau-Ponty influenced another philosopher whose writings have informed our thinking: Michel Foucault. Foucault is associated with the post-structuralist movement insofar as he questions the objectivity and stability of interpretative structures. Having attended Merleau-Ponty's lectures at the École Normal Supériure, he shares Merleau-Ponty's emphasis on the limits of language. His historical perspectives on madness and medicine reveal what he saw as the moral hypocrisy of modern medicine.

Foucault's understanding of "power-knowledge" has proved invaluable for our thinking (Foucault & Gordon, 1980). Arguing for the inseparability of the two concepts, he sees power not as a possession but rather as a pervasive force in everyday life. It is not merely repressive or constraining but often productive. For these reasons, we have found that it has deepened our understanding of psychoanalytic discourse.

It is in our attempts to better understand madness, a condition we consider to be a severe disorder of knowing, that integrating Merleau-Ponty's and Foucault's perspectives has proven useful. In her exploration of madness, Hanna Lyn Venable (2022), also draws on both. She integrates individual experiences of madness, which is in keeping with Merleau-Ponty's phenomenological approach, and the history of madness, supported by Foucault's "archeological" approach (see Chapter 6).

Let us now summarize the chapters on embodied relational knowing that you will find in this book.

In Chapter 1, "Lessons from the Adam and Eve Story." we have used the bible story, often referred to as "The Fall of Man," to introduce some of the ideas that we explore throughout this book. We begin by explaining that we were inspired to revisit the bible story when we came across Karl Ove Knausgaard's idea that, after eating from the tree of knowledge Adam and Eve became aware of one another insofar as, in his words, "all knowing is knowing in relation to the other" (Knausgaard, 2021). The idea that knowledge is always shared—with words and without them—lies at the heart of our concept of embodied relational knowing.

Of the many analysts who have identified the human quest for knowledge as the central theme of the Adam and Eve story, we have found that Lewis Aron's (2005) understanding most closely resembles our own. We examine Aron's comparison of the exegeses of the story by Erich Fromm and Rabbi Joseph Soloveitchik.

Later in the chapter, we distinguish our ideas about embodied relational knowing from the concept of meaning as elucidated by Robert Stolorow and his collaborators (e.g. Orange, Atwood & Stolorow, 1997/2001) as well as from Jessica Benjamin's (2018) "recognition theory." We explain how embodied relational knowing intersects with "I," "you," "we" and "world," the body-based words that describe what we believe are the components of human attention. We conclude with a clinical example that centers around both Doris's and her patient's embodied relational knowing needs.

Chapter 2, "Needing Not to Know or be Known," opens with our exploration of traumatic dissociation in relation to the need not to know. While a traumatic experience may register on a bodily level, we may lose access to any awareness that the experience occurred on a cognitive level. This discrepancy, we believe, often lies at the heart of what has been called "dissociation." Memory, we suggest, is always affected by both our needs to know and not know.

We emphasize that what many traumatized individuals need most not to know on a conscious level is anything that increases their experience of uncertainty. Rather than focusing on traumatic dissociation, however, we suggest that the need not to know is ubiquitous in human relationships, nowhere more so than in analytic relationships. Analysts, we believe, as well as patients, have needs not to know certain things about themselves and others—including their patients.

We examine the similarity between the need not to know and what Atwood and Stolorow term the "prereflective unconscious" (Atwood & Stolorow, 1980, 1981). The powerful effects of secrets as expressions of the need not to be known is addressed with reference to Kathryn Zerbe's (2019, 2025) work on the subject.

We provide an illustrative clinical example that centers around one of Jon's patient's needs not to know aspects of himself and the way it intersected with similar needs experienced by Jon. In another example, one of Doris's analytic relationships illustrates how the experience of shame often accompanies the need not to know or be known. The chapter concludes with an examination of the need not to know with respect to "I," "you," "we" and "world."

We devote Chapter 3, "Knowing Dreams," to the various ways in which certain dreams represent the interplay between the needs to know and be known and the needs not to know and not to be known. We compare Freud's idea of a dream's manifest and latent content (Freud, 1900) as well as Atwood and Stolorow's (1980, 1981) concept of the prereflective unconscious with our understanding. By way of illustration, we provide examples of our own dreams following the death of a parent as well as one by a member of our supervision/study group. We also provide examples of dreams that reveal progress in understanding our analytic relationships, dreams that anticipate patients' readiness to change, so-called "anxiety dreams," and dreams involving analysts and patients.

"Knowing Power," is the title and focus of Chapter 4. We examine Michel Foucault's (Foucault & Gordon, 1980) ideas about the inseparability of power and knowledge, particularly with respect to the analytic relationship. We emphasize Foucault's understanding of the positive uses of power—notably his disagreement with Freud and Reich over society's power to repress sexuality. Foucault's appreciation of the ways in which power is embodied is very much in keeping with our understanding on the bodily basis of knowing. We discuss his concept of "confession" and its relation to psychoanalytic therapy.

We also show how Joseph Lichtenberg's (2024) notion of power as animating all motivational activity and his evocative description of power as an experience of "can-do" and of being "a doer doing" is also supportive or our view.

We devote a portion of the chapter to a consideration of the ways in which power involves experiences of envy. We suggest that this sort of envy usually inhabits the realm of the need not to know. We describe sources of the need not to know including shame, which is often experienced with respect to envy as well as psychological stratagems for not knowing our envy of power. Efforts to "become" the envied other through imitation is an example.

While we believe that power dynamics are to be found in all our therapeutic relationships, we end the chapter by describing the ways in which power affected our work in very different ways with two of our patients.

In Chapter 5, "Knowing Love and Hate," we examine what may be among the most challenging aspects of psychoanalytic relationships: experiences of love and hate between analysts and patients. We ask whether it is possible to experience what Plato called the "divine madness" of love without also experiencing hate.

We begin by examining the connection between knowing and loving with respect to the perspectives of many well-regarded thinkers such as Wilhelm Reich (1933/1941), Erich Fromm (1956) and Ludwig Binswanger (cited in Frie, 1997) and Roger Frie (1997). We also discuss Heinz Kohut's (1984) assertion that object love is similar to selfobject experience insofar as both may strengthen one's sense of self.

While the patient's love for the analyst, the so-called erotic transferences, have been thoroughly investigated, few analysts have given accounts of their love for their patients. We discuss Jodie Messler Davies' (1994) exploration of this realm and her understanding of the longing to be loved for one's uniqueness. Even more rare are accounts of analysts' sexual feelings for their patients. We offer two clinical examples in which these feelings were prominent: in one the analyst's sexual desire was brought into the analytic dialogue and in the other it remained unverbalized.

We then turn to the issues of sex and gender and highlight Judith Butler's (2024) understanding that gender pertains to "a felt sense of the body."

Our discussion of hate begins with a portion of Freud's letter about his understanding of hatred and destructiveness in response to Albert Einstein's inquiries (Freud, 1932). We then present Ian Suttie's (1985) vehement disagreement with Freud's formulations. We also review discussions of analytic hatred by Donald Winnicott (1949) and Sue Grand (2024).

We end the chapter by presenting two examples involving hate in our analytic relationships. In Jon's example, experiences of hate between him and a patient were related to opposing political viewpoints. In Doris' example, the competitiveness of the publishing world served as a background for the development for hatred. Even more relevant was the effects of the patient's intense idealization of Doris on both analytic partners and its devastating dissolution.

In Chapter 6 we use the perspective of embodied relational knowing to examine what we call "disorders of knowing." We begin by describing our perspectives on obsessive-compulsive disorder (OCD), which we developed upon finding a common thread in the accounts of several OCD sufferers: their symptoms seemed to represent activities undertaken to reduce anxiety related to feelings of unbearable uncertainty. We provide numerous examples in which the development of patients' obsessive and compulsive symptoms seem to have been trauma related.

We then explore the possibility that patients who some self psychologically informed analysts regard as narcissistic and "mirror-hungry" might be understood as having unmet needs to be known. Doris's clinical example illustrates that for some patients, the need to have negative aspects of themselves known and accepted is as important as the recognition of what they value in themselves.

The need to know is often highly developed among patients who learned to "read" the nonverbal messages of caregivers and consequently prioritized their needs over their own. Jon's clinical example involved a patient whose need to serve other matched his own.

We outline a new approach to treating these patients with a variation of the embodied supervision approach we describe in Chapter 9 that involves asking patients to focus on their own embodied reactions and those of others.

We then describe how we use our perspective in working with patients with more severe forms of disorders of knowing—specifically dementia and madness. Starting with dementia patients and referencing the work of Mark Freeman (2021a,2021b), we describe the many clinical challenges we experienced in relation to the profound effect they had on our needs to know and be know as well as our needs not to know or be known. Doris's clinical example involves a patient suffering from Alzheimer's disease while Jon's example involves a patient who had experienced a severe brain injury. In both examples we emphasize how verbal communication was replaced by embodied forms of knowing and being known.

Our efforts to understand what we prefer to call "madness" in terms of its effects on the relational knowing worlds of patients perceived of as mad and those who are connected to them have been influenced by the extraordinary writings of George Atwood (2011), whose phenomenological contextualist approach allowed him to reject a view of psychosis as a medical disease. Instead, his clinical work reveals how the traumatic loss of human connectedness gives rise to the relational manifestations that are deemed psychotic. We also describe the influence on our work by the neuroscientific and phenomenological work of Vittorio Galese, Martina Ardizzi and Francesca Ferroni (2024) and Daniel Posner's (2025) as well as Hanna Lyn Venable's (2022) approach which involves integrating the philosophical perspectives of Merleau-Ponty and Foucault.

We present Jon's treatment of a patient diagnosed as schizophrenic who continually reported what seemed to be delusional and paranoid experiences. Although she would accept alternative ways of understanding her experience in Jon's presence, she would quickly revert to her idiosyncratic interpretations. Jon describes learning to accept her way of being in the world and how his witnessing of her experience meets her intense need to be known. We offer an understanding of her alternating experiences of herself in terms of alternations between her need to know and need not to know.

"Knowing Couples" is the title of Chapter 7. Viewing our therapeutic work with couples through the lens of embodied relational knowing has allowed us to better understand the reasons they seek our help and has enabled us to become more adept at helping them. We describe the intense need to know and be known at the beginning of most couples' relationships and suggest that the need not to know may be just as strong.

Since the bodies of couples communicate in very intimate ways, we have found that employing an embodied approach to therapeutic work with them has facilitated the process. We explain a variation of the approach that derives from our model of embodied supervision.

Secrets held by members of a couple sometimes come to be disruptive. In the opening clinical example, Jon describes his work with a couple after the woman's disclosure of her pre-marital sexual relationships to her husband created much distress. The secrets of both spouses were found to have little to do with her sexual experiences.

Differences in racial, class, or ethnic backgrounds also pose problems for couples. Doris provides an example in which the cultural pressures in the wife's family required them to move to the home of her ailing parents. The problems that emerged for the couple involved the perceptions held of them by members of their families of origin. We also give an example in which illness of one spouse was a significant factor.

While all our embodied relational knowing needs are influenced by our embeddedness in familial, cultural, ethnic, religious, professional and friendship communities, some of these communities serve to promote our development and healing while others are extremely detrimental to our wellbeing. We begin Chapter 8, "Knowing Communities" by discussing the benefits of such organizational communities as Alcoholics Anonymous (AA) and provide a clinical example of a patient who joined AA following a life-threatening illness related to his addiction.

We then describe how psychotherapy groups may function as knowing communities. In one example, Jon recounts his work with a patient in a group that he led that was inspired by both the approach developed by Albert Pesso (Pesso & Crandell, 1991) and Moreno's (1946) psychodrama. The patient's experience of being witnessed by the group allowed him to understand what had led him to seek help from others who were unavailable. Doris then describes some examples of therapeutic change within a long-standing psychotherapy group she has led.

Next, we examine the catastrophic effects of knowing communities that take the form of cults. We refer to the People's Temple cult led by Jim Jones in Guyana (Guinn, 2017). Our explanation of the power of these leaders involves the way they exploit the need to know and be known of their followers. We compare cult leaders with the fascistic rulers in today's world.

We then discuss dominating fathers in some families who behave much like fascist leaders. Doris provides an example of a patient who experienced her father as the all-knowing leader to her own detriment.

The chapter ends with a consideration of cult-like psychotherapy and psychoanalytic groups. We discuss Freud's overbearing leadership style and his intolerance for dissent.

In Chapter 9, "Knowing Supervision," we examine the effects of adding questions about needing to know and not know to the embodied supervision model we developed in our 2023 book. We demonstrate how these additions enhance supervisees' appreciation of the ways clinical knowledge and authority reside mainly in their bodies and those of their patients rather than in the theory or clinical experience of the supervisor. It also enables them to confront the limits of their ability to know their patients and themselves.

We begin by reviewing our 2023 model of embodied supervision and then explain how questions related to embodied relational knowing are introduced. We explain that in the **"I"** position, the supervisee is asked "What do you want to know about your patient? What do you want your patient to know about you? What don't you want to know about your patient? What don't you want your patient to know about you?" The same questions are then repeated in the "**you**" position except that they are asked of the patient whom the supervisee has "become" though imitation. We mention how the other members in the group form a knowing community that both supports the supervisee and provides new ideas for the development of the therapeutic process.

The remainder of the chapter is devoted to examples of embodied relational knowing supervision. The Zoom sessions of the group were recorded and transcribed which allowed us to use the actual words spoken by the supervisees. However, we altered the transcriptions to protect the confidentiality of patients and supervisees.

In the first example, the supervisee sought supervision because he had experienced himself as having lost the capacity to work with his patient. In the second example, the supervisee needed help managing a severely traumatized patient's intense needs for contact between sessions. Other accounts involved a "stuck" relationship, one in which the patient believed he was a "psychopath," a patient who made excessive demands for contact with her therapist, and one involving a patient's physically harming her child.

Each example includes comments by group members who both witness the supervisees' challenges with their patients and demonstrate that alternative understandings are possible.

Embodied relational knowing needs become greatly intensified in times of societal upheaval. In Chapter 10, "Knowing World," we examine the ways in which the need to know and be known are experienced, almost simultaneously, with the need not to know and be known during horrific world events. We find support for our understanding in the writings Dori Laub and Nanette Aurhahn and Roger Frie. We present Sue Grand's thought-provoking questions that were evoked by what she calls "Frie's ethical/familial/cultural predicament. We also describe Michelle Goldberg's opinion piece about the knowing-not knowing confusion that surrounded the infirmity of Joe Biden, the former U.S. president.

After suggesting that silence allows for the merger of knowing and not knowing, we present Thato Letsati's (2025) discussion of silence in relation to the exploration of racial trauma as well as Roger Frie's discussion of silence in the face of societal violence.

Noting that analysts as well as patients must be helped to find ways to talk about world conflicts and upheavals, we offer statements and excerpts from the writings of leading analytic thinkers that not only include their suggestions about ways to break their silence but some that also involve calls to action. We offer Donna Orange's writings on climate justice, Maxwell Sucharov's account of Canda's ongoing genocide of indigenous peoples, Ilene Philipson's thoughts on the ways in which analysts have displaced the "vitriol, binary thinking, moralism, and certitude that dominate our current, political landscape" onto analytic institutions, Stacy Berlin's thoughts on how to voice conflicts around sex and gender, Lynne Jacobs' calls to gently hold our humility to avoid ignoring the disquieting feelings associated with racial injustice, and Daniel Goldin's ideas about using pragmatic psychoanalysis to incorporate culture into analytic dialogues.

The chapter ends with Mark Freeman's answers to the following questions related to embodied relational knowing with respect to the world: What do you want to know about the world? What do you not want to know about the world? What do you want the world to know about you? What do you not want the world to know about you? What do you suspect you both want to know and not know?

In Chapter 11, "Beyond Knowing," we first consider what analysts are not able to know about themselves and their patients. It is not only that we cannot know how our relationships with new patients will develop, but there is much that we cannot know about those we have known for many years.

We then turn to the intriguing lure of what has been called "the uncanny." We re-examine Freud's 1919 paper on this realm in which he focused on the gruesome tale of the Sandman. We discuss John Zilcosky's (2016) suggestion that there was much Freud needed not to know about the horrors of World War I and his feelings about his sons who fought in it. We speculate that Freud's need not to know may have added to his turn away from his initial trauma hypothesis.

Our consideration of the uncanny phenomenon known as "the Doppelganger" in which one encounters a version of themselves in another person follows. We reflect on Freud's understanding of Doppelganger experiences in relations to what he may have needed not to know. We then examine Naomi Klein's understanding of 'the evil twin." Doris provides a clinical example involving an interracial couple. Next, we take up Klein's (2023) book about her nightmarish experience of being mistaken for Naomi Wolf, a woman whose political views were diametrically opposite her own. The chapter ends with a consideration of the us-them binary and societal Doppelgangers.

We conclude the chapter and our book with our thoughts on the importance of recognizing that an essential aspect of our work as analysts involves the humble acceptance that much about ourselves, our patients, their suffering and our efforts to help them lies beyond our knowing.

References

Aron, L. (2005). The Tree of Knowledge: Good and Evil Conflicting Interpretations. *Psychoanalytic Dialogue.*, 15: 681–707.

Atwood, G. E. & Stolorow, R. D. (1980). Psychoanalytic Concepts and the Representational World. *Psychoanal. Contemp. Thought*, 3: 267–290.

Atwood, G. E. & Stolorow, R. D. (1981). Experience and Conduct. *Contemporary Psychoanalysis*, 17: 197–208

Benjamin, J. (2018). *Beyond Doer and Done to: Recognition Theory, Intersubjectivity and the Third.* New York & London: Routledge/Taylor & Francis Group.

Brothers, D. & Sletvold, J. (2023a) Brothers, D. & Sletvold, J. (2022). Talking Bodies: A New Vision of Psychoanalysis. *Psychoanalytic Inquiry*, 42(4): 289–302. https://doi.org/10.1080/07351690.2022.2059292

Brothers, D. & Sletvold, J. (2023b). *A New Vision of Psychoanalytic Theory, Practice and Supervision: TALKING BODIES.* London and New York: Routledge Taylor & Frances Group.

Brothers, D. & Sletvold, J. (2023c). Foreign Bodies: The Risks and Rewards of Relational Knowing. Paper presented at the Psychology and the Other Symposium, October 7, 2023.

Buber, M. (2003). *Martin Buber's I and Thou.* Kennerth Kramer.

Butler, J. (2024). *Who's Afraid of Gender?* New York: Farrar, Straus & Giroux.

Freeman, M.P. (2021a). The Mother of Beauty: Death, Dementia, and the Face of the Divine. Presentation at the Psychology and the Other Conference. Boston, MA.

Freeman, M.P. (2021b). *Do I Look at You with Love? Reimagining the Story of Dementia.* Rotterdam & Boston: Brill/Sense.

Freud, S. (1915). The Unconscious. Standard Edition, 14: 166–204.

Frie, R. (1997). *Subjectivity and Intersubjectivity in Philosophy and Psychoanalysis: A Study of Sartre, Binswanger, Lacan, and Habermas.* Roman and Littlefield.

Frie, R. (2017), Not in My Family: German Memory and Responsibility After the Holocaust. New York: Oxford University Press.

Foucault, M. & Gordon, C. (1980). *Power/Knowledge: Selected Interviews and Other Writings, 1972-1977.* New York: Pantheon Books.

Fromm, E. (1956). *The Art of Loving.* New York: Harper & Brothers.

Gadamer, H. G. (1992). *Truth and Method.* New York: Seabyry Press.

Gallese, V., Ardizzi, M., & Ferroni, F. (2024). Schizophrenia and the Bodily Self. *Schizophrenia Research*, 269, 152–162.

Habermas, J. (1972). *Knowledge and Human Interests.* Trans. J.J. Shapiro. New York: Beacon Press.

Hoffman, E. (1999), The New Nomads. In A. Aciman, (Ed.) *Letters of Transit.* New York: The New Press, pp. 35–64.

Knausgaard, K. O. (2021). *The Morning Star.* London: Penguin, Random House, UK.

Kohut, H. (1971). *The Analysis of the Self.* New York: International Universities Press, Inc.

Kohut, H. (1977). *The Restoration of the Self.* New York: International Universities Press, Inc.

Merleau-Ponty, M. (1962). *Phenomenology of Perception*. Trans. Colin Smith. London: Routledge & Kegan Paul.

Moore, R. (1999). *The Creation of Reality in Psychoanalysis: A View of the Contributions of Donald Spence, Roy Schafer, Robert Stolorow, Irwin Z. Hoffman, and Beyond.* Hillsdale, NJ: Analytic Press.

Moreno, J. L. (1946). *Psychodrama: Foundations of psychotherapy*. (Vol. 1) Beacon, NY: Beacon House.

Nietzche, (1887/2017). *The Geneology of Morality*. Trans. Carol Diethe, .Ed. K. Ansell-Pearson Cambridge University Press.

Orange, D.M., Atwood, G. E., & Stolorow, R. D. (2001). *Working Intersubjectively: Contextualism in Psychoanalytic Practice*. London & New York: Routledge, Taylor and Francis Group.

Orange, D. M. (2003). The Creation of Reality in Psychoanalysis: A View of the Contributions of Donald Spence, Roy Schafer, Robert Stolorow, Irwin Z. Hoffman, and Beyond. By Richard Moore. *Psychoanalytic Review*, 90: 303–309.

Pesso, A., & Crandell, J. (Eds.) (1991). *Moving Psychotherapy*. Brookline Books.

Reich, W. (1972). *Character Analysis* (3rd ed.). Trans. V. R. Carfagno. New York: Farrar, Straus and Giroux. (Original work published 1949.)

Ricoeur, P. (1970). *Freud and Philosophy: An Essay on Interpretation*. New Haven, Ct.: Yale Unversity Press.

Stänicke, E. Zachrisson, A., & Vetlesen, A.J. (2020). The Epistemological Stance of Psychoanalysis: Revisiting the Kantian Legacy. *Psychoanal Q.*, 89(2): 281–304. https://doi.org/10.1080/00332828.2020.1717229.PMID: 35312457

Stolorow, R. D. (1988). Transference and the Therapeutic Process. *Psychoanalytic Review*, 75: 245–254.

Stolorow, R. D., Atwood, G. E., & Brandchaft, B. (1988). Masochism and Its Treatment. *Bulletin of the Menninger Clinic*, 52(6): 504–509.

Winnicott, D. W. (1965). *The Maturational Process and the Facilitating Environment: Studies in the Theory of Emotional Development* 64: 37–55.

Zerbe, K. (2019). The Secret Life of Secrets: Deleterious Psychosomatic Effects on Patients and Analysts. *Journal of the American Psychoanalytic Association*, 67: 185–214.

Zerbe, K. (2025). *Secrets in Psychotherapy: Stories that Inform Clinical Work*. ISBN: 9781003471578

Zilcosky, J. (2016). *Uncanny Encounters: Literature, Psychoanalysis, and the End of Alterity*. Northwestern University Press.

1 Lessons From the Adam and Eve Story

What could psychoanalysts today possibly find of value in the Old Testament of the Bible? Before we began our exploration of the seemingly endless complexities of what we have come to call "embodied relational knowing," we would have been hard pressed to point to anything in the old bible stories that we thought might be relevant to our work. Taken literally, these tales are full of contradictions and absurdities. Then, by some serendipitous coincidence we came across an account by Karl Ove Knausgaard (2021), a prolific Norwegian novelist, of the biblical story in Genesis 3 of The Old Testament, commonly known as "The Fall of Man".

According to Knausgaard, when Adam and Eve ate from the tree of knowledge, they immediately became aware of one another insofar as all knowing is knowing in relation to the other. While we believe that knowledge of being "I" is "prereflective," that is, it does not originate in the context of mirroring by others (Frie, 1997), we are convinced that we could not develop our knowledge of ourselves in isolation. Moreover, since we are utterly dependent on one another to survive both physically and psychologically, it makes sense that, after becoming aware of one another, these first humans would want to know as much as possible about the other, and that they would want the other to know them.

What we explore in this book starts with the idea that, throughout our lives, we need to be known by others and to know them. It is only through our efforts, however unfulfillable, to realize these needs (often experienced as longings)—that we gain knowledge of ourselves. Embodied relational knowing takes into account that our lives are embedded within relationships with others who also need to be known by us and who need to know us. Just as complexly intertwined as the needs and longings for relational knowledge, are our needs not to know and not to be known—needs that often, but not always, result from traumatic experiences (See Chapter 2). And at certain times, the needs to know and not know converge, sometimes because what we know in an embodied way is unavailable to our cognitive ways of knowing. All of the these reciprocal needs, as we hope to demonstrate, lie at

DOI: 10.4324/9781003487883-2

the heart of the spoken and unspoken dialogues that occur within psychoanalytic relationships.

On reading "The Fall" for ourselves, we discovered references to much that you will find in the pages of this book. We soon realized that making sense of the story depends on appreciating its metaphorical rather than literal meanings. As we hope will become clear, relational knowing makes use both of verbal language—often in the form of metaphors—and, to a large extent, nonverbal language that is communicated by what we have called "talking bodies" (Brothers and Sletvold, 2023a). Once the literal meanings of the bible stories are replaced with metaphorical meanings, they no longer seem absurd.

Before trying to explain what we found of value in the Adam and Eve tale, let us review how it is written in the bible. The main characters in the story are God, the man (Adam), the woman (Eve) and the serpent. The narrative begins with the serpent asking Eve if it is true that God has told them not to eat of the fruit of any tree in the garden. Eve says that they may eat of the fruit of all the trees in the garden but for one. Of its fruit God has said: "Ye shall not eat of it, neither shall ye touch it, lest ye die." The serpent tells her they will surely not die, for God knows that the day they eat of the fruit their eyes will be opened and they will become as God, knowing good and evil. Eve eats of the fruit, as does Adam. The first thing that happens is that they discover they are naked, whereafter they hide themselves from God, who, on finding them and realizing what has happened, banishes them from the garden of Eden (The New Oxford Annotated Bible, 1977).

Few readers would need to question what made Eve susceptible to the serpent's inducement that she acquire knowledge. Being human is virtually synonymous with wanting to explore, examine, understand, know. One has only to observe healthy babies for a few minutes to notice their intense urge to find out everything they can about their surroundings by means of sight, hearing, taste, smell and touch. They are keen observers of the human and nonhuman world around them. Clearly knowing does not depend on having verbal language. But as soon as healthy babies gain words, they ask question after question. They are quick to use language to find out about the world they find themselves in. It seems likely that this trait had enormous evolutionary value and contributed to the survival of our species. We are convinced that our psychological survival as individuals depends on what we call embodied relational knowing.

We are hardly the first analysts to become interested in the Adam and Eve story. It has served as a veritable Rorschach test for many psychoanalysts (e.g. Aron, 2005; Bodin, 2010; Bouchard, 1996; Fodor, 1954; Fromm, 1966; Gilligan, 2020: Lederer,1964; Osman, 2000). They have each highlighted aspects of the story that most closely jibes with their theoretical bent.

Bouchard (1996), who mentions the similarity of the story to the myth of Oedipus, notes that a number of analysts from various psychoanalytic schools have focused on one key element in the story: the human quest for knowledge. Much as we too explore the longing to know and to be known in this book, our interest in the story differs considerably from the many ways in which the analysts mentioned by Bouchard have examined knowing. To give some examples: they have variously discussed "intellectualism" as a means of coping with unresolved sexual conflicts, to obtain the narcissistic gratification of omniscience and omnipotence, and as a reflection of problems with separation/individuation. They have described the inability to tolerate not knowing in terms of problems at oral, anal-sadistic, and oedipal stages of development, and as problems in the early mother–child relationship.

Although there is undoubtedly a great deal to be gained from all the psychoanalytic readings of "the Fall," Lewis Aron's (2005) take on it most closely corresponds to the one that we examine in this chapter, namely how the story explicates relational connectedness. In his article, Aron compares the different exegeses of the story by Erich Fromm and Rabbi Joseph Soloveitchik to show the implications of each interpretation on such issues as autonomy and relatedness, assertion, and submission, will and surrender, and obedience and rebellion.

Aron applauds Fromm's "radical humanistic" reading of the bible and the Eden story. He points out that, for Fromm, the Christian interpretation of the story obscures its clear meaning. Much, for Fromm, has to do with Adam's rebellion (eating the fruit from the tree of knowledge despite God's warning) for which God punished him by expelling him from Eden. As Fromm notes: "His (Adam's) first act of disobedience is the beginning of human history, because it is the beginning of human freedom" (Fromm,1966, p. 23, parenthesis added). He contends that the human being is "beset by the existential dichotomy of being within nature and yet transcending it by the fact of having self-awareness and choice. Man creates himself through the first act of freedom—the freedom to disobey—to say 'no'."

For Aron, Fromm's reading of the story goes too far in emphasizing the human striving toward freedom and independence. Soloveitchik's exegesis, Aron asserts, resonates more closely with his own views concerning mutuality and interdependence. Soloveitchik, according to Aron, emphasizes the changed account of Adam (Adam I) in the first version of Genesis, which represents him as part of nature, "an object among objects," to the second version (Adam II) in which he is represented as "a human person, who lives in a relational framework requiring passion, love, and companionship." In line with Soloveitchik's account, Aron describes Adam II as struggling with two sets of fears: the fear of death and the fear of ignorance. "Man," he says, "wants to love and to know."

We see the longings to love and to know as inextricably intertwined (see Chapter 5). In fact, for us, loving is impossible without some form of knowing. We find support for our position in Fromm's popular book The *Art of Loving*, published in 1956. In it he describes love as an art that requires knowledge and skill. He writes:

> Man is gifted with reason; he is life being aware of itself; he has awareness of himself, of his fellow man.
>
> (Fromm, 1956, p. 6)

According to Fromm, this awareness leads us to understand our separation and isolation from one another and the world and confronts us with the fearful idea that we will die. Although we agree that humans have struggled mightily to come to terms with the inevitability of death, in contrast to Fromm, we do not see our embodied awareness of ourselves and one another as necessarily leading to a sense of separation and isolation. Rather, for us, knowing and being known—the aspects of knowledge that correspond most closely to relational experience—lead to a deepening sense of what we call "we-connectedness."

One reason that the quest for relational knowing is so pervasive in human life is that each human is unique and, to some extent, unknowable. Even identical twins are distinctly different from one another. Our encounters with the unknowable uniqueness of each human being serve to intensify our longings to be known by others and to know them and open us to others' needs to be known and to know.

We do not mean to suggest that we are completely impenetrable to one another and that we can never feel deeply known by others or that we never deeply know others. We are convinced that the sense of being known and knowing is integral to loving relations (see Chapter 5). However, even in close, loving relationships, knowing is subject to disruption and imperfection.

When the limits of our ability to know ourselves and others are taken into account, the idea that empathy is the only way for analysts to know their patients comes into question. We consider the use of empathy to have been a necessary antidote to the traditional analytic stance of knowing based on the analysts' theoretical understanding. Our experiences suggest that much empathic connectedness to others can be achieved by tuning into our bodily reactions to them and by means of embodied imitation. Yet, we feel it is important to heed Heinz Kohut's understanding that empathy cannot be assumed to be perfect, it always proceeds by trial and error.

Empathic knowing, we believe, is limited to the extent that it is based mainly on sameness, or finding oneself in the other as Kohut's (1971, 1977) term "vicarious introspection" suggests. In other words, by assuming along with Harry Stack Sullivan that "we are all much more simply human than otherwise" (1946–1947) we attempt to know the other's experience by stepping into the shoes of the other and looking inward. Knowing based on an awareness of difference and unknowability is quite different. Since our unique humanness cannot be fully grasped by means of vicarious introspection, our longing to be fully known, despite its poignant intensity, can never be completely met. Moreover, since much of our own experience is unavailable to consciousness, we cannot know ourselves completely either.

We believe that attempts by clinicians to connect to patients empathically should guide their practices but that when these attempts are tempered by the realization that they must fail to some extent, room is left for surprise, novelty and fresh insight. We have also contended that knowing based on the limits of empathy makes for more ethical analytic relationships (see Brothers and Sletvold, 2023c). As Kohut made clear, understanding the effects of failures in empathy both by patients' early caregivers as well as by their analysts is crucial to therapeutic healing. To the extent that empathy is rarely perfect or complete, longings to be known by others, to know others and not to know or be known are evoked.

Let us return to "The Fall." We find it significant that, after eating from the tree of knowledge, Adam and Eve immediately became ashamed of their nakedness. We suspect that, to some extent, this aspect of the story reflects the need to hide sexual desire. After all, it is hard to keep naked bodies from revealing sexual arousal. Erich Fromm (1956) disagrees that it was the nakedness of their bodies per se that gave rise to shame for Adam and Eve. He suggests that their nakedness revealed their separateness. He writes:

> *The awareness of human separation, without reunion by love—is the source of shame. It is at the same time the source of guilt and anxiety.*
>
> (Fromm, 1956, p. 9)

However strong the link between nakedness and shame, we believe that shame is ubiquitous in analytic relationships. We address these considerations in Chapter 2.

Meaning and Embodied Relational Knowing

You may have already suspected that relational knowing bears some resemblance to what others have called "meaning." In the famous memoir of his experiences at Auschwitz, *The Search for Meaning,* Victor Frankl (1946) asserts:

> Ultimately, man should not ask what the meaning of his life is, but rather must recognize that it is he who is asked. In a word, each man is questioned by life; and he can only answer to life by answering for his own life; to life he can only respond by being responsible.
>
> (Frankl, 1946, p. 109)

We find these words reminiscent of Fromm's assertion that man is "life being aware of itself" (see above). Frankl suggests that meaning is to be found in faith in god and in love. Drawing on his own experience, he asserts that the salvation of man is through love and in love. As we discuss in Chapter 5, the relationship between loving and knowing often occupies our therapeutic relationships.

Robert Stolorow is an analyst who has demonstrated the centrality of meaning in many of his own publications, as well as in quite a few of those he has co-authored with others (see, e.g., Orange, Atwood & Stolorow, 1977; Stolorow, Brandchaft and Atwood, 1988). In a 2016 article written with George Atwood, meaning is described as follows:

> From our vantage point, therapeutic inquiry is a dialogical process in which each participant, in varying degrees and at different times, engages in reflection upon three interrelated domains—the meanings organizing one's own experience, the meanings organizing the other's experience, and the dynamic intersubjective system constituted by these interacting worlds of meaning. Furthermore, in this dialogical process each participant (far from entering the other's subjective world and leaving his or her own outside) continually draws on his or her own experiential world in search of analogues for the possible meanings governing the other's experiences. Empathic (introspective) understanding is thus grasped as an emergent property of a dialogical system, rather than as a privileged possession of an isolated mind.
>
> (Atwood & Stolorow, 2016, p. 106)

We find Atwood and Stolorow's understanding of "interacting worlds of meaning" in psychoanalytic inquiry to be similar to our understanding of the complex intertwining of the I-you-we-world flow that organizes human relating (Brothers & Sletvold, 2023a, 2023b). However, we believe that it neglects an essential aspects of knowing: embodiment.

Relational knowing is profoundly embodied. It is not only babies who use nonverbal means to learn about others, we continue to do so all of our lives. We constantly use our own bodies to inform us about the feelings, attitudes and wishes of important others. We could not know anything about others without our bodily sensing of them. Nor could they know us without their bodily sensing of us.

Insofar as the concept of meaning refers mainly to cognitive understanding, it cannot address those times when knowing is experienced in an embodied way but what is known is not available to cognitive comprehension. That is, there is a discrepancy between what is known bodily and what is known cognitively. We also believe that Stolorow's (1988) understanding of meaning as "an indivisible amalgam of cognition and affect" (p. 246) ignores what Jon Fosse, the 2023 Nobel Prize winner in literature, calls "the unsayable." In an online 2023 *Guardian* article Chris Power quotes Fosse as commenting:

> I often say that there are two languages. The words that I wrote, the words you can understand, and behind that there's a silent language. And it's in that silent language that the real meaning may lie.
>
> (Powers quoting Fosse, October 28, 2023, *Guardian*)

In the interview, Fosse adds: "It's only in the silence that you can hear God's voice. Maybe." Where Fosse finds the divine, we locate embodiment. We do not mean to suggest that spirituality has no place in embodied relational knowing, but we will leave that realm to others who are better acquainted with it. What we do feel more able to discuss is how the body speaks the unsayable. Referring to what Norwegian poet, Helge Torvund, called "the silence between the words,' we have suggested it is in these spaces that "bodies do much of their talking" (Brothers & Sletvold, 2023a, p. 16).

The therapeutic situation for Stolorow depends on the analysts' grasp of what he calls patients' "organizing principles." In a March 21, 2012, online interview by Eric Maisel on *Psychology Today*, he explains this concept as follows:

> Developmentally, recurring patterns of emotional interaction within the child-caregiver system give rise to principles (thematic patterns, meaning-structures, cognitive-emotional schemas) that shape subsequent emotional experiences, especially experiences of significant relationships. Such organizing principles are unconscious, not in the sense of being repressed, but in being prereflective. Ordinarily, we just experience our experiences; we do not reflect on the principles or meanings that shape them. The totality of a person's prereflective organizing principles, from my perspective, constitutes his or her character.
>
> (Maisel, *Psychology Today*. March 21, 2012)

While we believe that identifying recurring patterns of relating may be useful for analysts who hope to fulfill their patients' longing to by known, we object to the extent to which organizing principles are disembodied and seemingly impervious to the messages within the embodied context of the person's surround.

Recognition Theory and Embodied Relational Knowing

There is much overlap in our understanding of relational knowing and Jessica Benjamin's theory of recognition. According to Benjamin (2018):

> Recognition as an organizing idea may be thought of in two ways: first, as a psychic position in which we know the other's mind as an equal source of intention and agency, affecting and begin affected, and second as a process of action, the essence of responsiveness in interaction.
>
> (Benjamin, 2018, p. 3)

Contrasting intersubjective psychoanalysis with original psychoanalytic theorizing, she notes:

> Conceiving an intersubjective psychoanalysis means positing the presence of two knowing and not-knowing subjects in the room—each one potentially engaged in recognition of the other's alterity, the other's different center of perspective, or perhaps equally unsettled and engaged in avoiding that recognition.
>
> (Benjamin, 2018, p. 3)

An important concept for Benjamin, is "the Third." She defines it as "a position in which we impliciltly recognize the other as a 'like subject,' a being we can experience as an 'other mind' " (Benjamin, 2018, p. 21). Breakdown of recognition, she notes, "occurs when the two sides of sameness and difference, congruence and incongruence fail to be upheld by the crossbeam of the third." The breakdown spells collapse into what she calls "two-ness." Benjamin charts the growth of "the third" in early development through the movement between recognition and breakdown, and shows how it parallels the enactments in the psychoanalytic relationship. She illustrates how acknowledgment promotes healing in both individual and social trauma.

Benjamin's "second meaning of "recognition," pertains to expressive behaviors that

> confirm that I am seen, known, my intentions have been understood, I have an impact on you, and this must mean that I matter to you. And reciprocally that I see and know you, I understand your intentions, your actions affect me and you matter to me.
>
> (Benjamin, 2018, p. 21)

In contrast to Benjamin's ideas about recognition, our understanding of embodied relational knowing places even greater emphasis on the impossibility of being known completely or knowing others completely. She mentions that the psychoanalytic relationship is made up of two subjects each of whom is potentially engaged in recognition of the other's alterity. Although we subscribe to the potential for the recognition of alterity by the analytic couple, we emphasize the innumerable ways in which the recognition of the other's alterity is likely to be countered by needs and longings to be completely known by the other and to know the other. Moreover, Benjamin's understanding, like Stolorow, leaves little room for the times when knowing and not knowing either converge or are discrepant.

Subscribing to the ideas advanced most notably by Emmanuel Levinas (1961) about the irreducible alterity of each person, we do not assume that we can ever completely know what is on another person's mind. It is just the irreducible alterity of human beings, we contend, that gives rise to needs for increasingly complex forms of relational knowing that change over the course of development and in response to changing analytic contexts. Our approach is distinguished by our emphasis on the ongoing nature of analytic engagements that reflect longings to know and be known, not to know and not to be known, and their intersection.

In addition to Levinas, we find support for our approach in Frie's (1997) examination of the work of Ludwig Binswanger for whom intersubjectivity is always marked by differences among individual subjects. Binswanger, who draws on Buber's conceptualization of I-Thou relations as the basis for love, insists that love always includes the potential for breakdown. These inevitable breakdowns and the longings they inflame, we believe, profoundly influence relationships throughout our lives and suffuse our analytic relationships.

We see the earliest roots of longings for relational knowing in the stranger anxiety shown by 8 or 9-month-old babies. They become distressed when those they have known in innumerable nonverbal ways appear to have been replaced by others who are unknown to them. We suspect that the hostility shown to foreigners, which is especially virulent in relation to migrants in today's world, stems, at least in part, from these early experiences. While object relations theorists have suggested that "object constancy" is attainable by children 2 or 3 years old, by which they mean that they are able to maintain a stable and consistent perception of others even when they are out of sight, we do not believe that this ability signals the end of longings to more fully know others and to be known by them.

Consequently we contend that recognition, as Benjamin defines it, to the extent that it is based on the realization of alterity, is rarely, if ever, sustained. Like Benjamin, we too believe that experiences of we-connectedness are likely to alleviate the sense of aloneness that haunts our lives. These experiences may be intensely pleasurable—even blissful—especially in the context of love, yet they are constantly vulnerable to disturbance. We are continually reminded of terrifying moments of not being known or knowing others particularly when undergoing a fresh trauma or when these experiences are revived in current life (see Chapter 2). Indefinitely sustained experiences of we-connectedness marked by mutual recognition are not available to most of us, with the possible exception of those who devote their lives to extreme forms of spiritual practice.

In summary our understanding of relational knowing differs from recognition theory insofar as we place more emphasis on the unknowable, unwordable, embodied aspects of connectedness and our appreciation of the entanglement and disentanglement of the needs to know and be known and the needs not to know or be known.

Embodied Relational Knowing in Our Time

We believe that the development of the internet and the growing importance of social media greatly affects the meanings we glean from our interactions with others in terms of relational knowing. Consider one conspicuous way in which the quest to be known is manifested in today's world. Thanks to the popularity of social media platforms, making ourselves known to others has never been undertaken with more zeal and efficacy. Posting images of themselves on social media that reveal the minutia of their lives, thousands of people exhibit the way they dress, the food they eat, the entertainment they enjoy, and the company they keep. Many seem intent on conveying that they are enjoying enviable lives of satisfaction, fulfillment and well-being. What they seem bent on hiding are their inadequacies and misfortunes.

At times the need to be known seems to be so intense that being known by only a few others does not suffice. Such a need seems to lead certain people to create glorifying myths about themselves. We have almost become used to the lies told by politicians, notably the twice elected US president, Donald Trump and other politicians who greatly inflate their achievements.

A recent book, *The Collaborators*, by Ian Baruma (2023), describes three people who created fabulous narratives about themselves that were widely believed to be true. Felix Kersten, masseur to Heinrich Himmler and others in the Nazi elite; Yoshiko Kawashima, the dispossessed Manchu princess who spied for the Japanese; and Friedrich Weinreb, the "fixer" whose fellow Jews paid him to secure reprieves from deportation to concentration camps, and were instead betrayed to the German secret police, publicly cast themselves as saviors, serving noble causes and saving lives.

The tendency to accept lies by politicians and other powerful figures in the world also reflects the ways in which we need not to know others, particularly if knowing what has been lied about prevents us from glorifying these figures. How we experience ourselves as we shall soon attempt to explain depends on how we are known by others.

The need to know others which, we believe, is as intense and pervasive as the need to be known, also seems to be heightened in today's world. A visit to any bookshop or newsstand or social media site will reveal how the need to know others has been catered to and, at times, exploited in Western societies. From thoroughly researched biographies in scholarly books to the latest film star scandal in gossip magazines, the demand for details about the lives of others has been big business. While acquiring knowledge about a famous person's life undoubtedly serves to enhance one's own sense of self though some form of vicarious identification, we believe that the need to acquire such knowledge must also derive from the survival value of knowing those upon whom one's very sense of individuated selfhood depends.

Relational Knowing as Story-Telling

We are convinced that we all spin stories about ourselves and that these stories, which are both verbal and nonverbal, constitute that ways in which we know ourselves and others. Our stories may either inflate or deflate our worthiness and may confirm or refute how we have come to be known by others in our early lives. And, as we attempt to demonstrate in the clinical examples throughout this book, analysts expend a great deal of effort to sift through these stories. We believe that, in the course of analytic relationships, both patients and analysts develop stories about themselves and one another that allow them to make better and better sense of their lives. Doing so allows for an increasingly fluid flow of attention among the complexly interacting components of "I," "you," "we" and "world."

But it is not just what is happening in the world at any given moment that informs relational knowing. What has happened in the past is equally, and at times, more significant. Our own experiences in a world that is ever-changing, as well as the world that our ancestors lived in, greatly affect how we know ourselves and others. The past and present world also affects our longings for embodied relational knowing. We suspect that one reason for the powerful draw of fiction, plays, dance performances etc. resides in the opportunities they provide for us to know ourselves and others as we exist in our world.

How We Know "I," "You," "We" and "World"

We believe that using the words, "I," "you," "we" and "world" makes for more body-based communication than using such traditional psychoanalytic terms as "ego," "the self," "object," "object relations," "the field" and "the third" (Brothers & Sletvold, 2023a, 2023b). We proposed that most of human experiencing involves a flow of attention among the various components of what we consider the I-you-we-world totality. We further explained that the complexity of the I-you-we-world flow is compounded insofar as the experience of I-you-we-world in one individual is continually affected by and affects the experience of I-you-we-world of all of the individual's relational partners. We now hope to show that while there is no way to isolate the individual components of the I-you-we-world flow, since each component illuminates different aspects of embodied relational knowing, we now examine them separately.

Knowing "I"

Since Socrates declared that the unexamined life was not worth living and advised humans to know themselves, this counsel has been repeated through the ages. Nevertheless, philosophers hold extremely varied positions on how we know ourselves. Analytic philosophers such as Donald Davidson (1991), Gilbert Ryle (1949) and Daniel Dennet (1991) have attempted to reduce subjective experience, which includes self-knowledge, to states of immaterial minds or automata, while postmodern philosophers have attempted to deconstruct the subject such that all aspects of human psychology are socially determined.

Roger Frie (1997) has taken exception to the idea that consciousness can be reduced to the cognitive model of reflection. Self-consciousness, Frie notes, is grounded in "being-familiar-with oneself" that is, prior to all reflection. He asserts that "self-acquaintance precedes relation" (p. 11). He draws on Binswanger, Sartre and Frank who, in various ways, take exception to Heidegger's (1927/1996) assertion that that human existence is understandable only as "being-in-the-world." While supporting Heidegger's opposition to Descartes' cogito, Frie disagrees with Heidegger's assertion that self-consciousness is not initially given, but is derived through Dasein's projection as being-in-the world. Frie writes:

> The difficulty with this approach to the familiarity of the self with itself lies in the use of a reflexive model to clarify the structure of subjectivity.
>
> (Frie, 1997, p. 49)

In stating his own position, Frie writes: " . . .the I that is made present in the act of reflection must be the result of a prior familiarity of self" (p. 59). In addition, Frie suggests that the irreducible nature of prereflective being-familiar-with-oneself makes the intersubjective relationship possible. We would say that "prereflective being-familiar-with-oneself" is what underlies the quest to be known and to know others. For us, being familiar with oneself involves a nascent sense of knowing one's own thoughts and feelings—even if that knowing is imperfect and incomplete. In early life this knowing is mainly body-based and nonverbalizable. It is this pre-reflective knowing that sets the stage for our need to be known by others and to know them. Although we pre-reflexibly know ourselves it is only in interaction with others that our worded and unworded narratives about ourselves develop.

It is now widely accepted by contemporary analysts that it is within the give and take of relationships with caregivers that the child develops the sense of I. The idea that one can know oneself by simply focusing one one's own experience in isolation has been thoroughly debunked. Infant researchers like Daniel Stern (2000) and Beatrice Beebe (2014) by micro-analyzing videos of parent–child interactions, have greatly refined our understanding of the ways in which nonverbal communicative modes including gaze, gestures, sounds, etc. affect self development. We believe that longings to be known and to know others, to the extent that such longings inevitably meet with disappointments in parent-child interactions—even if these disappointments are not traumatizing—begin to take shape in the earliest interactions between the child and caregivers.

It seems to us that the ways in which people come to know just what they mean when they start a sentence with "I" is a process that changes continually throughout the life span. Rather than being a fixed awareness, one's knowledge of "I," which we believe is always manifested in the form of narratives, subtly changes according to one's relational surround and all that is experienced within it.

When parents and others fail to provide children with responsiveness that adequately reflects their unique humanness, their quest to be known may come to dominate their lives and, if they enter psychoanalysis, to organize the dynamics of embodied relational knowing between them and their analysts.

As our clinical examples will hopefully demonstrate, the ways in which this occurs is endlessly varied. To get a sense of the enormous variability, think of patients who have developed a narrative of themselves as "good," well-behaved and obedient children. We suppose that their caregivers greatly influenced the development of this narrative by indicating verbally and nonverbally that they will be available to them only to the extent that they conformed to this way of being. How this narrative becomes known in the analytic situation is extremely variable. For some patients, the hope to be fully known prompts them to become "bad" patients by missing sessions, coming late, failing to pay bills on time or maintaining that their therapists are unhelpful. For others who are so completely convinced that they will be rejected if they reveal the slighted indication of being less than "good", they become model patients who keep their darkest fears and feelings to themselves.

Knowing "You"

Children learn very early in their lives that their psychological survival depends in part on how well they are able to know their parents and caretakers. Children devote themselves to their quest to know these important figures by careful observation and, perhaps even more importantly, through imitation. We know that moments after birth, infants can imitate facial expressions and they become increasingly skilled at copying the bodily movements of those around them. Through observation and imitation they learn what feelings, attitudes, beliefs, language, even what kinds of music and artwork is acceptable to their parents and which are not. They also learn what they should not know about themselves and others. Words may never be used to communicate this information.

It probably goes without saying that analysts become a powerful "you" for their patients. But they are no exception to the human need for relational knowing and their patients become important "you" figures for them. Freud seems to have ignored his own need to be known as well as his patients' need to know him by positioning himself behind patients who were required to recline on couches. The idea that analysts only need to know their patients without regard for their patients need to know them has created considerable distress for both analytic partners. We now understand that although the early analysts were not in their patients' line of vision during sessions they were by no means unknown. Analysts reveal much about themselves simply by the way they speak, the silences and pauses in their speech, subtle movements in their chairs, the ways they walk and greet patients, etc.

We suspect that analysts often give silent messages to patients that they should not be known by them. These messages are perceived in many ways that depend on a patient's relational history. For some patients, it is as if analysts exist in a rarified plane above theirs, and therefore, that they are too godlike to be approached. These patients may experience shame for their arrogance in wanting to know their analysts and for longing to decrease the enormous gap separating them. For others it is a challenge to find out everything that their analysts go to great lengths to hide. Analysts, these patients assume, like the Wizard of Oz, are essentially untrustworthy. Just, as is true of every aspect of the analytic exchange, the variations on this theme are endless.

But what do analysts need to be known about themselves? While there are probably as many answers to this question as there are analysts, we suspect that most analysts wish to be known as caring professionals, who are well-versed in the art of healing. When patients fail to grasp this, analysts are likely to experience a storm of emotions (More about this in Chapter 4 in which we discuss power and knowing).

Knowing "We"

Perhaps, the most poignant of all experiences of being known and knowing others is captured by Buber's (1970) conception of I-thou relations. Contrasting I-thou with I-it, Buber notes the I-thou can only be spoken with the whole being and is characterized by mutuality, openness and directness whereas I-it lacks these qualities. But as he points out, an I-thou relation can never be sustained indefinitely, so that a I-it relation inevitably follows.

Buber contends that I and Thou are encompassed together and enter into a symmetrical relation in which the identification of the I and the identification of the Thou are reciprocally generated. As Frie has written in his discussion of Buber:

> The between is found neither in the I nor in the thou but only as that which has its being between them. The between exists only in relation, and is not continuous, but is reconstituted with each new human encounter. The between denotes the reality of relation.
>
> (Frie, 1997, p. 91)

For us, the idea that what exists between I and Thou is "reconstituted with each new human encounter" captures how relational knowing is continually transformed in the analytic encounter. It is just this renewal that makes the ongoing process of narrative development healing for both analytic partners. As patients and analysts become more fully known to one another, all of their relationships tend to become richer, more complex and more complete.

It is probably simultaneous with developing a sense of oneself and others that a sense of "we" develops in early life. As Daniel Stern (2000), Beatrice Beebe (2014) and other infant researchers have made clear, it is the infant's interactions with others from the beginning of its life that enables the emergent sense of self with which it is born to develop. Infants keen abilities to observe and imitate allow them to join in the bodily communication that provides a sense of belonging in all of the overlapping relational systems in which their lives are embedded. However, we believe the safety and ease the child experiences from we-connectedness is not consistently sustainable. The need to be known and to know others within the complex relational systems that comprise one's we-experience are stirred by inevitable disturbances within these systems. Societal traumas both present and past severely disturb one's sense of we-connectedness. But much less severe disturbances may stir these longings.

Knowing "World"

Although we emphasize the unknowable uniqueness of each human being we by no means dispute the idea the we live in a shared world. Being incompletely known is not equivalent to living in isolation. We are in full agreement with Binswanger and Frie (1997, p. 132) who assert that while human development is grounded in linguistic dialogue, language does not create the existence of world; it is the manifestation of prior world disclosure. In fact linguistic communication is possible only because we live in a shared world.

At the same time, it is our inseparability from world as it affects how we know "I," "you" and "we" that profoundly affects our needs to be known and to know others. It is hardly news that humans have always lived in a traumatized and traumatizing world. We contend that trauma, as we shall try to explain in the next chapter, profoundly affects the way we know one another and our need not to know and be known. Moreover, our clinical experience suggests that experiences of embodied relational knowing are transmitted intergenerationally; they reflect the ways in which traumatic experiences during wars, political strife and natural disasters affected the embodied relational knowing of our ancestors.

Our unfulfilled needs and longings to be known and to know others often results in a sense of "homesickness," or the feeling of not belonging in the world (Brothers & Lewis, 2012). We long for what Hans Gadamer described as "heimat," a German term that resists translation, that refers both to home and homeland. According to Gadamer (1992) "heimat," which alludes to an experience so stable and reliable, it precedes all knowing and deciding, is inextricably linked to language. Sigmund Freud confirmed this observation by suggesting that what the emigrant feels so "particularly painfully" is . . . "the loss of the language in which one had lived and thought, and which one will never be able to replace with another for all one's efforts at empathy" (Gay, 1988, p. 632). And, although Heinz Kohut spoke only English at home after emigrating to the United States, he noted that he felt really content only when he could "speak and think German," his native language (Cocks, 1994, p. 10).

Describing the predicament of emigrants, who, for a time, may be without language, Eva Hoffman (1999, p. 48) underscores how much a sense of self depends on having "a living speech within us." "To lose an internal language," she observes, "is to subside into an inarticulate darkness in which we become alien to ourselves."

When children fail to experience a sense of belonging in the world, they invariably come to see themselves as inadequate and unworthy. For some this leads to a burning desire to be seen in a positive light. At times this desire becomes so great that it can only be met through the accomplishment of extraordinary feats of daring and creativity. These efforts are undertaken not just for the sake of recognition but also for the sake of fame, even notoriety. To be widely known, even as someone who causes harm to others, can powerfully motivate those whose connections to others has depended on their being the "bad" child.

While we believe the aspects of relational knowing affect every psychoanalytic relationship, it was particularly prominent in the relationship we now describe.

Doris and Eva

When I met Eva for the first time about 20 years ago, the issue of analytic disclosure had become a hot topic in psychoanalytic circles. Eva, an attractive, 40-year-old, married white woman, tested my stance on the issue almost from the start. "Do you live in this building or just work here?" "I love those earrings, where did you get them?" "You mentioned that you'll be away next month, where are you going?" These are just a sampling of the questions she routinely asked.

Despite the discomfort I sometimes experienced in revealing these details about myself and my life to her, I sensed that if I wanted to help Eva, I would have to answer her questions as honestly and completely as I possibly could. Although she had never suggested that our connectedness depended on these exchanges, I believe that she communicated the urgency of her need to ask and to be answered without words through the tensions in her body, her facial expressions and subtle changes in the tone of her voice. My appreciation of the importance of both her asking me questions and my giving her answers has only deepened over time. And what I did not even suspect when we first met was how much I would learn about my own need to know as a result.

Eva's life was pockmarked with unanswered questions: What happened to her half-siblings after they disappeared during her childhood? Why was her father away from home so much of the time and where did he go? What made her mother so clearly prefer her younger brother? And perhaps, most daunting, how did her father die? Her mother had once claimed that Eva had killed him since he suffered a heart attack following a dinner in which Eva had argued with her mother. Although she was only nine years old at the time, Eva had been left alone with him during his final moments, a deeply traumatizing experience.

Eva's mother often responded to her questions by saying, "It's none of your business" or when she did answer a question, it was often with a blatant lie. Shortly after her father's death, Eva fell mute. She remembers being unable to speak for several weeks but could not imagine what had prevented her from expressing herself in words. We have recently wondered if, had she spoken, might she have felt compelled to contradict her mother's version of what happened to her father. To have done so would have put her at risk for being physically abused (her mother had often hit Eva with little provocation) or, even worse, for being met with silence. During such times, Eva felt herself shrink into terrifying states of non-existence.

In addition to becoming mute, Eva seems to have needed not to know what happened during long periods of her childhood. Her blankness included the birthday parties her mother said she had made for her, Christmas celebrations, and anything beyond a few scant memories of being with her father. In one memory she is waiting outside the house for him to come home from work, but how he greeted her eludes her recall.

Much of the content in the early years of our work centered around her relationship with her daughter. Having lost all contact with her own mother, Eva could not free herself of the dread of an intergenerational repetition. The slightest misunderstanding between her and her daughter filled her with terror. Eve believed that the basis of her closeness with her daughter was their mutual knowing of one another. When her daughter left for college and formed close relationships with peers, Eva, grief-stricken, lamented, "I just don't know her anymore."

As our relationship deepened, the voice that Eva used for questioning me changed greatly from how it sounded during her earlier fact-finding inquiries. Speaking in the voice of a very young child, she would ask me for explanations about herself and events in her life that I believed she was far better equipped to give than I. However, sensing the intensity of her need, I would answer as simply and directly as I could, as if I really were speaking to a young child. Although Eva did not seem to "become" a young child in every other respect, I wondered if the change in her resembled the experience of people suffering from dissociative identity disorder who create alter personalities.

Much as Eva questioned me about herself and me in the manner of a lost child, I discovered that she prided herself on her expertise about everything having to do with illnesses and remedies for them. Having suffered from a variety of gastrointestinal maladies herself, she had learned all that could be known about them and disclosed her knowledge in a highly authoritative way. When her husband's genetic condition became apparent, she researched every aspect of his illness. Unfortunately, she would then inform him about which doctors to consult to and what remedies to try with great certitude about the infallibility of her opinions. His obstinate refusal to follow her advice suggested that he experienced her as trying to control him with her claims to superior knowledge. He would viciously respond to her with vulgar and insulting comments, apparently intending to silence her. She would tearfully describe feeling hurt and angered by his refusal to accept what she believed to be her sound medical advice.

We have since come to understand that, for Eva, only incontrovertible facts about a given subject could be accepted as the truth. Since she had been unable to distinguish between her mother's truthful statements and her lies, she relied on her own ability to search for authoritative answers to her questions, often involving prolonged and thorough research. Her greatest gift, she felt, was to offer to others what she had learned through her painstaking investigations of the facts—especially when they involved medical or scientific studies. To have her offerings of "truth" rejected was not only deeply wounding, it threatened her sometimes tenuous sense of reality.

Eva seemed to experience my initial efforts to explore the hostile exchanges between her and her husband as insensitive attacks—especially when I asked her to imagine what had led him to react with such hostility. Didn't I see how stupid he was not to follow her carefully researched advice, she asked. I decided to abandon these efforts for a time for fear of repeating her mother's failures to confirm her experience of truth.

Our relationship changed considerably as Eva gradually began to answer her own questions instead of relying on me to do so. No longer sounding like a child, but like the self-assured woman she was becoming, she would offer feeling-laden explanations of the situations involved. It was shocking for me to discover that I missed the pleasure I derived from answering her questions. On reflecting about what had been pleasurable in giving my admittedly superficial answers to Eva, I realized how similar we were in this respect. I too had learned not to ask questions of my own mother for fear that I would not be able to determine their truthfulness. And like Eva, I had compensated for this lack of trustworthy guidance by becoming a truth seeker myself. Although my expertise was not in medical knowledge but psychological theory, I realized that my pleasure resulted partly from the sense of power dispensing my carefully researched truths afforded me. As the one with the answers, I no longer experienced the powerlessness I endured as a child. However, my pleasure and sense of empowerment came at the cost of a cherished belief—that my analytic encounters were meetings between "foreign bodies."

Although I had not engaged in a verbal power struggle with Eva, I wondered if the power I derived from answering her questions had somehow been communicated to her bodily. Is that why she rebuffed my initial efforts to explore her confrontations with her husband, I wondered.

It was only when I was able to connect with my own need to be the one who knows and to appreciate the power position this afforded me, that I became able to address Eva's situation in a way that she could tolerate. I suggested to Eva that since she had needed to rely on herself for answers, providing proven medical information might have compensated her for a needed but absent experience in her development. Silently acknowledging that I could not know the best way for Eva to communicate with her husband, must have changed the way she experienced me. I believe that she felt freer to find her own way to deal with his need for medical information.

My awareness of my similarity to Eva with respect to relational knowing subtly changed our relationship. Although it was never verbally communicated between us, Eva and I connected in a more collegial way that allowed for more humor and playfulness. I believe that Eva benefitted from realizing that her need to know was not necessarily a source of friction and rejection in her other relationships. She seemed to have become less likely to insist on the rightness of her advice-giving and to allow for greater mutuality in her interactions with others.

While Doris's relationship with Eva centered around both of their needs to know, there was much that they needed not to know about themselves and one another. Eva needed not to know that there could be flaws in her medical knowledge and that her efforts to inform her husband about them were damaging their relationship. Doris needed not to know her similarities to Eva as an expert knower. In the next chapter we examine the need not to know in greater detail.

References

Aron, L. (2005). The Tree of Knowledge: Good and Evil Conflicting Interpretations. *Psychoanalytic Dialogue*, 15: 681–707.

Atwood, G. E. & Stolorow, R. D. (2016). Walking the Tightrope of Emotional Dwelling. *Psychoanalytic Dialogues*, 26: 103–108.

Baruma, I. (2023). *The Collaborators: Three Stories of Deception and Survival in World War II.* New York: Penguin Random House.

Beebe, B. (2014). My Journey in Infant Research and Psychoanalysis: Microanalysis, a Social Microscope. *Psychoanalytic Psychology*, 31: 4–25.

Beebe, B. & Lachmann, F. (2002). *Infant Research and Adult Treatment.* Hillsdale, NJ: Analytic Press.

Benjamin, J. (2018). *Beyond Doer and Done to: Recognition Theory, Intersubjectivity and the Third.* New York & London: Routledge/Taylor & Francis Group.

Bodin, G. (2010). Expulsion from the Garden of Eden. *Scandinavian Psychoanalytic Review*, 33: 96–105.

Bouchard, M. (1996). The Need To Know and the Inability To Tolerate Not Knowing. Blema S. Steinberg. pp. 85-103. *Psychoanalytic Quarterly*, 65: 672–673.

Brothers, D & Lewis, J. (2012). On Homesickness, Exile, and the Self-Psychological Language of Home-Coming. *International Journal of Psychoanalytic Self Psychology*, 7: 2, 180–195.

Brothers, D. & Sletvold, J. (2023a). *A New Vision of Psychoanalytic Theory, Practice and Supervision: TALKING BODIES.* London and New York: Routledge Taylor & Frances Group.

Brothers, D. & Sletvold, J. (2023b) Talking Bodies: A New Vision of Psychoanalysis. *Psychoanalytic Inquiry*, 42(4): 289–302. https://doi.org/10.1080/07351690.2022.2059292

Brothers, D. & Sletvold, J. (2023c). Foreign Bodies: The Risks and Rewards of Relational Knowing. Paper presented at the Psychology and the Other Symposium, October 7, 2023.

Buber, M. (1970). *I and Thou.* Trans. W. Kaufmann. New York: Charles Scribner.

Cocks, G. (1994) *The Curve of Life: Correspondence of Heinz Kohut 1923-1941.* Chicago: The University of Chicago Press.

Colman, W. (1988). After the Fall: Original Loss and the Limits of Redemption. *Free Associations*, 1: 59–83
Davidson, D. (1991). Three Varieties of Knowledge. *Royal Institute of Philosophy Supplement*, 30: 153–166. https://doi.org/10.1017/S1358246100007748.
Dennett, D. C. (1991). *Consciousness Explained*. New York: Little, Brown and Co.
Fodor, A. (1954). The Fall of Man in the Book of Genesis. *American Imago*, 11(2) 203–231.
Frankl, V. E. (1946). *Man's Search for Meaning*. Beacon Press.
Frie, R. (1997). *Subjectivity and Intersubjectivity in Philosophy and Psychoanalysis: A Study of Sartre, Binswanger, Lacan, and Habermas*. Lanham, Maryland: Roman and Littlefield.
Fromm, E. (1956). *The Art of Loving*. New York: Harper & Brothers.
Fromm, E. (1966). *You Shall Be as Gods: A Radical Interpretation of the Old Testament and Its Tradition*. New York, NY: Holt, Rinehart and Winston.
Gadamer, H. G. (1992). *Truth and Method*. New York: Seabyry Press.
Gilligan, C.N. (2020). Disrupting the Story: Enter Eve. *Journal of the American Psychoanalytic Association*, 68: 675–693.
Gay, P. (1988). *Freud: A Life for His Time*. New York: Norton. New York: Harper & Row.
Hoffman, E. (1999). The New Nomads. In A. Aciman (Ed.), *Letters of Transit*. New York: The New Press, pp. 35–64.
Heidegger, M. (1927/1996). *Being and Time*. Trans. J. Stambaugh. New York: New York State University Press
Knausgaard, K. O. (2021). *The Morning Star*. London: Penguin, Random House, UK.
Kohut, H. (1971). *The Analysis of the Self*. New York: International Universities Press, Inc.
Kohut, H. (1977). *The Restoration of the Self*. New York: International Universities Press, Inc.
Lederer, W. (1964). Oedipus and the Serpent. *Psychoanalytic Review*, 51(4): 79–102.
Levinas, E. (1961). *Totality and Infinity An Essay on Exteriority*. Duquesne University Press.
Maisel, E. (2016), Robert Stolorow on Emotional Trauma and Psychoanalysis, Psychology Today. *Psychology Today* blog: www.psychologytoday.com/blog/feeling-relating-existing
Orange, D. M., Atwood, G. E., & Stolorow, R. D. (1997). *Working Intersubjectively: Contextualism in Psychoanalytic Practice*. Hillsdale, NJ: Analytic Press.
Osman, M. P. (2000). The Adam and Eve Story as Exemplar of an Early-Life Variant of the Oedipus Complex. *Journal of the American Psychoanalytic Association*, 48: 1295–1325.
Powers, C. (2023) Online Interview of Jon Fosse. *The Guardian*, October 28, 2023.
Reich, W. (1972). *Character Analysis* (3rd ed.). Trans. V. R. Carfagno. New York: Farrar, Straus and Giroux. (Original work published 1949.)
Ryle, G. ([1949] 2002). *The Concept of Mind*. Chicago: University of Chicago Press. p. 327.
Steinberg, B. S. (1993). The Need To Know and the Inability to Tolerate Not Knowing. *Canadian Journal of Psychoanalysis*, I(2): 85–103.
Stern, D. N. (2000). *The Interpersonal World of the Infant: A View From Psychoanalysis and Developmental Psychology* (2nd ed.). New York: Basic Books.

Stolorow, R. D. (1988). Transference and the Therapeutic Process. *Psychoanalytic Review*, 75: 245–254.
Stolorow, R. D., Atwood, G. E., & Brandchaft, B. (1988). Masochism and its treatment. *Bulletin of the Menninger Clinic*, 52(6), 504–509.
Sullivan, H. S. (1946–1947). *Lectures on the Interpersonal Theory of Psychiatry*. Washington School of Psychiatry.
Sullivan, H. S. (1953). *The Interpersonal Theory of Psychiatry*. New York: Norton.
The New Oxford Annotated Bible (1977). (M. Coogan & M. Brettler, Eds.) Oxford: Oxford University Press.
Wellington, A. (2009). *The Philosophy of F H Jacoby*. Wentworth Press.

2 Needing Not to Know or Be Known

Contemporary analysts are no longer amazed to find that many patients who have undergone traumatic experiences are unable to say much about what happened to them or even whether anything happened at all. It has become usual to understand this loss of memory in terms of dissociation, generally understood as the disconnection of aspects of traumatic experiences such that they are often lost to consciousness.

We (Brothers & Sletvold, (2022, 2023)]. have suggested that dissociation functions to reduce the complexity of lived experience, which concomitantly reduces the person's sense of unbearable uncertainty that we find to be the hallmark of trauma. We mentioned the tendency toward black and white thinking and the creation of binaries as complexity-reducing dissociative strategies that make traumatized individuals feel more certain. We also suggested that complexity and uncertainty are reduced when emphasis is placed on one of the components of the I-you-we-world flow (Brothers & Sletvold, 2023). The traumatized person may then be experienced as I-centered, you-centered, we-centered or world-centered. We have assumed that dissociation in the context of trauma is usually unavailable to consciousness—at least until it is worked through in treatment.

By considering dissociation from the perspective of embodied relational knowing, our understanding has deepened and become more complex. What is often dissociated in the context of trauma is a person's bodily sense of knowing about a traumatic experience. You might say that our bodies always know when we have experienced trauma. On a conscious cognitive level, however, the traumatized person may not know that the experience occurred. It is not remembered.

We understand the disregard for what we know bodily and the failure of memory in traumatic circumstances as a consequence of the intensification of the need not to know. It is often because it is just what traumatized people need not to know on a cognitive level that is experienced on a bodily level that their conscious sense of not knowing is strengthened. It might be said that, in the context of trauma, knowing and not knowing co-exist.

DOI: 10.4324/9781003487883-3

Much that occurs within analytic relationships revolves around a patient's memories, no matter if the memory reported is about an experience that happened moments before the patient entered the analytic session or about one that occurred many years earlier. We find it clinically helpful to consider that a patient's need to know and remember as accurately as possible is constrained and complexified by the need not to know. As Roger Frie's (2017) courageous efforts to grapple with his family's experiences of the Holocaust reminds us, despite the painful struggle involved, we may come to better know the nature of remembering and forgetting by exploring our relational worlds in ways that take into account the intermingling of the personal, the familial, the cultural and the historical. We see this exploration as central to the therapeutic process.

Analysts are just as likely to need not to know about traumatic experiences on a conscious level as their patients. Unfortunately, when analysts' traumatic memories are revived in the analytic relationship, they may fail to recognize how their need not to know affects their patients' experience and the unfolding of the healing process. And just as analysts can learn what their patients need not to know in an embodied way, so patients sometimes learn what their analysts need not to know from bodily feelings. They may then go to great lengths to shield their analysts from unwanted knowing even if it compromises the healing process. For example, one of Doris's patients shielded her former analyst from having to confront her increasing dementia until the analyst could no longer remember what had transpired in their sessions.

Memory, as Roger Frie (2017) has demonstrated, is also profoundly affected by cultural and historical circumstances, and, we might add, by what one's family deems acceptable to remember.

We cannot be sure that any memory—even one that is registered on a bodily level—is accurate. If, as Bessel van der Kolk's book title proclaims, "the body keeps the score," we can never be sure if it is the correct score. We could not recall a body-based memory without the assistance of our cognitive processing and our cognitive processing is influenced by our needs to know and not to know.

Our clinical experience leads us to believe that the need not to know may be generated by experiences that are not necessarily traumatic. In fact, we see it as a pervasive aspect of being human and an important feature of analytic relationships. In this respect, the need not to know is somewhat like "the prereflective unconscious," one of the several forms of intersubjectively derived modes of consciousness described by Atwood and Stolorow (1980,1981). In describing the prereflective unconscious, which co-exists with "the dynamic unconscious" "the unvalidated unconscious," as well as "ontological unconsciousness" or the loss of one's sense of being, Stolorow (2006) observed:

> *The* ***pre-reflective unconscious*** *is* the system of organizing principles, formed in a lifetime of relational experiences, that pattern and thematize one's experiential world. Such principles, although not repressed, ordinarily operate outside the domain of reflective self-awareness.
>
> (Stolorow, 2006, p. 237)

Like the pre-reflectively unconscious, the need not to know, can often be made conscious when attention is focused on it. For us, however, the need not to know cannot be assumed to relate to a life-long experiential organization. While it may interfere with the complexly intertwined flow of "I," "you," "we" and "world," it sometimes reflects more fleeting, transitory experiences. Feeling safely involved in a trustworthy analytic relationship, what is known bodily may become available to conscious knowing.

Since trauma is, and has always been, ubiquitous in our world, it is possible that, if we were to search diligently enough, we might find remnants of trauma whenever the need not to know occurs. In contrast to the need not to know about traumatic experiences, we have found that the need not to know about other aspects of lived experience may be easily brought into conscious awareness. In the next chapter, we describe how this occurs when dreams are told in analytic sessions.

Therapeutic Relationships and the Need Not to Know

As our clinical example in Chapter 1 hopefully demonstrates, longings to be known and to know may dominate a therapeutic relationship. However, the needs of both therapeutic partners not to know or be known are often just as meaningful.

Analysts are just as likely to enter relationships not wanting to be known in certain ways and may even wish not to know some things about their patients—particularly when those things stir painful memories in their own lives. We discuss the power dynamics of not knowing in Chapter 3.

Secrets

"No mortal," Freud (1905) tells us, "can keep a secret. If his lips are silent, he chatters with his fingertips; betrayal oozes out of him at every pore." This assertion is very much in line both with Freud's sensitivity to bodily communication and his conviction that analysts can know the unconscious experience of their patients. Those who tried to keep secrets had violated the analyst's direction to say everything that comes to mind. Refraining from complete openness was considered in terms of resistance to the analytic processes, a way of avoiding the expression of sexual and aggressive impulses. In a successful analysis, the patient's resistances would be analyzed such that they were resolved.

In contrast to this perspective, we believe that virtually all adults have secrets. Even though the unspoken messages that pass between talking bodies are often unwittingly communicated, we do not feel that secrets are ever fully disclosed through embodiment. Since perception of these embodied messages is filtered through each individual's own subjectivity it is never completely clear that we have gained access to the other's experience (Sletvold, 2014). As we mentioned above, the score that bodies keep may be inaccurate.

It seems unlikely to us that any patient has ever fully obeyed the traditional analyst's "say everything that comes to mind" command. It seems more likely that most patients enter therapeutic relationships with a wish to keep aspects of themselves to themselves and that they are also likely to wish not to know some things about their analysts. They may want to keep their analysts from knowing things that might weaken their analysts' positive regard or even alienate or disgust them. Concomitantly, they may need not to know things about their analysts that would interfere with their longing for the analyst to heal them or provide missed experiences. While they may not always be aware of what they wish not to know or to be known about themselves, these aspects of their experience are usually available to consciousness if they are identified.

Kathryn Zerbe (2019, 2025) reminds us that keeping secrets is a developmental achievement for the child (Spitz, 1957, 1965; Winnicott, 1960) and suggests that not all secrets are unconscious or multi-layered. However, she provides examples of patients who assumed that their secret was irreparably destructive to an essential relationship with their therapists. She notes that shame, guilt, narcissistic vulnerability, unconscious identification with an injured party, and developmental deficit were other factors involved in keeping secrets from their analysts.

Analysts are ethically bound to keep secret much that they know about the lives of their patients to maintain confidentiality. Yet the analyst's secret keeping may take its emotional toll on the analyst's well-being. Zerbe (2025) refers to the work of Bok (1983) on the harmful effects of the analyst's secret-keeping. Bok gives examples in which she became aware of what she calls a patient's "corrosive secret" through her embodied countertransference.

We believe that the need to keep secrets by patients and analysts is just one of a vast array of reactions to the needs not to know or be known that saturate analytic relationships. In the following example, we highlight a patient's need not to know, how it changed, and how it affected his analyst.

Jon and Tom

During the early years of what had been a remarkably smooth therapeutic relationship, Tom had seemed strangely incurious about himself and me (Jon). Although we were both analysts, he had not asked me to say anything about myself, my family, my theoretical orientation or my feelings for him. I had first imagined that since he had been trained in a traditional Freudian institute where analysts are not expected to disclose personal information, his failure to ask about me was simply "following the rules." But then I realized that

I had not detected any bodily signs of his interest in my life or my feelings for him. His need not to know me appeared to be very strong.

I had no idea what had stopped Tom from asking himself—and me—about puzzling aspects of his life. Why, for example, had he chosen to remain in what we had discovered was a dreadful marriage? With prompting from me, he revealed that his wife, who struggled with severe mental disturbances, had abused him psychologically and physically. He initially attributed his reluctance to leave his wife to his concern for their daughter, even though she was nearly grown up.

It was when his daughter entered her own therapy and revealed to Tom that her mother had tormented her during psychotic rages that he began to awaken from his deep "sleep." As his willingness to know became increasingly urgent he re-examined his early assumption that he had married his wife because "we fell in love." He then spoke of his intense idealization of his wife's family. While he himself had a working-class background, his wife's father had been a prominent university professor and, even years after his death, had been viewed as a leading ethical figure by most of the family members. While aware that every one of this man's sons and daughters had struggled with emotional problems so severe that two had been placed in mental hospitals, including his wife, Tom had not questioned whether this revered man might have been a poor father.

A striking moment in our relationship occurred soon after Tom's daughter had asked him to participate in a family therapy session with his wife. The family therapist quickly ended the session because he felt that Tom's wife was so severely disorganized that the session might prove harmful. Although the session had ended quickly, it was not before his daughter had provided some striking details of abuse by her mother—both physical and emotional. Tom then said, "I had always imagined that I was a good father, but I had closed my eyes to the dreadful suffering my wife had inflicted on my precious daughter."

He then spoke about needing to see himself as a good child, a good student, and a good provider as well as a good father. He added, "I had always compared myself to others and found that I was somehow better than they were." Tom's realization about his self-perception as "the good child" helped me to understand how he had been blind to the hurtful aspects of his father-in-law's treatment of his family. Had he allowed himself to know about the dark side of his father-in-law, he might have also become aware of his own failings.

But it was not only Tom who needed not to know things about the dark side of life. It was also me. I had accepted Tom's "sleepiness" because, like Tom, it has been difficult for me to know about the hurtfulness of some of my relatives. I had not fully recognized Tom's need not to know because it was much like my own.

Around this time, I told Tom that I was reducing my patient hours and would be spending many months out of Norway each year, Tom then seemed to become increasingly willing to investigate areas of his life that had been simply accepted as "the way things were." Each session was filled with more information about his father-in-law that revealed him as anything but the ethical figure he had once admired. I considered the likelihood that Tom had hoped that by become such a good and interesting patient, I would not suggest bringing the analysis to a close.

Tom then began to wonder if not knowing about his wife's abusiveness and the unethical activities of his father-in-law were the very reasons for his need to stay connected to them.

In contact with them, he could somehow not know that he could be "bad." They, not he, were bad. His badness, he said, was a well-kept secret—a secret that he kept from himself as well. When this secret was broken, his understanding of himself and his world deepened.

Tom has recently become more and more interested in me and my work. He has expressed interest in my writings and has even asked why I now spent so much time out of Norway. It has only been since Tom has shown his wish to know me that I have been able to appreciate the extent to which I felt deprived by his lack of interest in me. I imagine that it felt shameful to admit—even to myself—that I had ever felt the need to be better known by him.

With these changes in our relational knowing, our sense of closeness as colleagues as well as therapeutic partners has increased. Our relationship is now more alive and vibrant than ever—and so is Tom.

Shame and the Need Not to Know

In our experience, the need not to know often accompanies anxiety about having the feelings that knowing or being known might generate. Shame, we have found, is chief among them. Even when we are not aware of feeling shame our bodies reveal its presence. There are countless ways in which shame is embodied. Some people sweat while others feel cold; some blush while others grow pale; some gesture effusively while others are still. When these bodily manifestations of shame reach our awareness, we often attempt to hide them from the eyes of others. Think of shameful patients who cover their faces with their hands or seem to fold in on themselves as if to protect their bodies from searching eyes. Still others use their clothing for cover. Countless newspaper photos show the turned-up collars and pulled down hats as those accused of crimes attempt to hide their bodies from view.

Culture seems to greatly affect the sensitivity to shame; the need to "save face" may be stronger in the East than it is in the West. Yet it's hard to for us to imagine a place where the tortures of shame are not profoundly embodied.

The link between the need not to know and shame is illustrated in a therapeutic relationship that Doris described as part of a chapter in her 2008 book, *Toward a Psychology of Uncertainty*. We offer a condensed version of what Doris called "The Shrug" that highlights a mutual need not to know.

Doris and Zoe

In the early days of our relationship, Zoe, an attractive, highly intelligent woman of 40, seemed not to perceive that I (Doris) had any imperfections or vulnerabilities. It had not occurred to me at the time to think about the meaning of her not wanting to know my flaws. Were there some flaws that she might be able to accept but not others? Was not knowing about another person's flaws a means of keeping safe?

She compared me very favorably to her previous therapist who, she said, had grievously injured her with lapses in his attention. But it was not long before our therapeutic honeymoon ended, and Zoe now "knew" with great certainty exactly what my therapeutic flaws were and reported them to me with biting disdain. I chose the wrong words, or uttered them with a discordant tone of voice, or failed to speak when she had hoped I would. Although we both suffered from the injurious aftereffects of my behavior which, we came to understand, re-opened wounds inflicted during her abusive childhood, I remained convinced that our work together would eventually prove healing.

On one fateful day, however, Zoe's pained expression let me know that I had committed an especially egregious error in relating. How could I have failed to return a phone message in which she had informed me of her father's death, she demanded. I explained that since she had been estranged from her father for many years and had not sounded particularly upset, I had not understood that she needed to hear from me right away. She replied that any responsible therapist would have known better than to have accepted her blasé manner at face value. After all, her father's abusiveness had affected every part of her life. Wasn't word of his death worthy of some notice on my part? What could I have been thinking?

After listening to her complaints for several minutes, I shrugged my shoulders. On reflection, I believe I meant to convey something like "Yes, I know I let you down, but, come now, my not calling you wasn't that big a deal." "You shrugged!" Zoe said, her voice dripping with contempt, "How could you!" But then, as if possessed by some particularly malicious demon, and hardly aware of doing so, I shrugged a second time. Although I made feeble apologies for having done this again, Zoe abruptly ended the treatment after stating that she could not work with someone who was so out of touch with herself.

It was only after a dream in which I welcomed Zoe into my office only to find it littered with broken glass, that I glimpsed what I had tried so hard not to know. For the first time, I connected my failure to return her call informing me of her father's death with what had been happening in my own life at the time. I had been terribly worried that the illness of a beloved relative would prove life-threatening. Now it occurred to me that I could not have returned her call without referring to her father's death in a way that would have stirred the fearful possibility that my relative might die. When, in that fateful session, she inadvertently called my avoidance into question, my shrug expressed the anger I could not feel, nor accept. I *had* intended my shrug to be hurtful!

As soon as I acknowledged my intention to inflict pain, Zoe's reactions began to make sense to me. I realized that by failing to admit my wish to hurt her, I had subjected her to what she had claimed was the worst part of her father's abusiveness. He had never taken responsibility for his actions but instead had blamed his vicious physical and verbal attacks on her provocations. How could she remain in treatment with someone who also disavowed her hurtfulness?

I had known that Zoe's mother had been neglectful and indifferent to her. But suddenly I realized that for Zoe, it was as if her mother had always responded to her needs with a bored shrug. To say that I was filled with shame at realizing how hurtful my shrug had been to Zoe and, even more, that I had actually meant to be hurtful, is an understatement.

Within days of these realizations, a strange, I would almost say, uncanny, thing occurred: Zoe and I found ourselves on the same bus, something that had never happened before. My greeting must have conveyed to her that I had changed. The next day she phoned me, "I'm doing much better," she said, "thanks to our work together. But I had to leave, didn't I?" I said that I thought I understood why she did.

When I think back to my relationship with Zoe, I realize that I had dissociated the bodily evidence of both my own shame and hers, thus mutually intensifying the need not to know. I now suspect that Zoe's criticisms of me following our initial "honeymoon" were her way of becoming the shamer rather than the shamed. As our relationship deepened, it must have taken very little for me to remind her of her father's hurtfulness and her mother's indifference. A distracted look, an offhand comment, the ringing of the phone—many little offenses must have proceeded the fateful shrug. But I had not only failed to become aware of the bodily signs of Zoe's shame, but I had failed to attend to my own. My anger and hostility were highly effective strategies for hiding shame from myself.

While Zoe and Doris were eventually able to resume a therapeutic relationship that was immensely healing for both, we have come to realize that knowing about one's vulnerability to shame in a particular clinical situation may not preclude experiencing shame in others.

There is no easy fix for shameful and shaming interactions. One reason for our continuing vulnerability to shame concerns the powerful role of memory. Shameful experiences with patients, either our own or theirs are likely to revive painful memories in which we were shamed in the past. It is not only our patients' memories of shame that affect their perception of us, but our own memories of being shamed that affect our perception of them. The interplay of these memories continually, albeit subtly, then affects what is going on from moment to moment in the clinical encounter.

Perhaps even more than declarative or verbal memories those that are implicit and nonverbal intensify shame in the clinical encounter. Just as

Beebe et al. (2014) have shown through micro-analysis of videos that the infant-caretaker exchange is affected by split-second changes in facial expression, duration of gaze, etc., so it is that fleeting implicit memories evoke and re-evoke shame in the therapeutic encounter.

The description of Doris's relationship with Zoe occurs in a chapter in her book that deals with the topic of burnout. While shameful experiences in themselves may well engender burnout, which is a devastating condition marked by feelings of unworthiness and inadequacy that have even led some to give up the healing professions, the need not to know about what spurred shame is probably equally responsible. Gaps in knowing created by our wish not to know about shame greatly affect our sense of embodied connectedness with others, our sense of "we" and the sense of embodied wholeness we derive from it, without which we are incapable of true empathy and compassion. We maintain that it is not too much empathy and compassion for our patients and ourselves that leads to burnout, but too little.

Our very humanness—our imperfect attunement and our inability to know others and ourselves completely—makes us exceedingly vulnerable not only to shame but to our need not to know about shame. Yet we believe that when shame is taken out of the shadows and allowed to enter the daylight of dialogue, our relationships are likely to grow and deepen.

The Need Not to Know and Blaming Others

Avoidance of shame is probably a factor in the experience of people who continually experience themselves as victimized by the hurtfulness of others as well as their environment. They present themselves as blameless and innocent in their interactions while needing not to know how their posture affects those around them. Naturally, the power dynamics within clinical situations are greatly affected as the clinical example of Jon and Bette in the next chapter illustrates.

The Need Not to Know "I," "You," "We" and "World"

In Chapter 1, we examined the need to know and be known in terms of the various components of the I-you-we-world flow. Now we look at the need not to know in the same way.

The Need Not to Know "I"

Almost from the moment we are born we begin to learn what we can and cannot know about ourselves if we are to become the children our caregivers need. Our psychological survival often depends on our ability not to know! We understand what we cannot know even before we learn to speak. It is communicated nonverbally by such means as touch, gaze, tone of voice, etc. Moreover, what should and should not be known about oneself and others is passed from one generation to the next and is greatly influenced by ethnicity and culture (Brothers, 2014).

So, for example, in highly gender-divided families and cultures, many boys need not to know that they possess qualities stereotypically associated with girls and most girls in these settings need to not to know that they are like boys. It may be that the bodily sense of being similar to members of the opposite sex intensifies their need not to know.

Some children need not to know that they resemble a relative who is detested. Others need not to know that they prefer calm and quiet when the family culture emphasizes noisy interaction. Still others need to not to know that they are more or less intelligent or good looking or caring than a preferred sibling.

Trauma is often discussed in terms of the traumatized person's victimization. The shameful feelings of helpless vulnerability to abuse or exploitation often generate dissociative not knowing. But as Doris's experience with Zoe suggests, the need not to know that one has inflicted pain, may be just as difficult to know. Such reactions have often been found among combat veterans (e.g. Ulman & Brothers, 1988). Similarly, incest survivors who have participated in sexual encounters with family members may need not to know about their own involvement, even when they had few opportunities to experience connectedness with anyone other than the incestuous abuser.

We are reminded of a colleague of ours, a 50-year-old white woman, who is a talented clinician, a caring wife and mother, and part of a close community of friends. Although few signs now remain, she struggled to find her calling as an analyst after a troubled adolescence and young adulthood marked by drug use and alcohol abuse.

As a very young child, she had learned not to know that she was at least as intelligent as her older siblings, if not more so. Her father would engage the older children in deep conversations about current events, history, literature, etc. When she tried to join them, she was teased and pushed aside. Her mother, with whom she was close, had little interest in developing her intellect. It was only after her parents had died, and she had entered analysis, that she discovered the only way for her to find a place in her family was not to know how smart she was.

The Need Not to Know You

A frequently encountered instance of not knowing occurs among children who cannot know that their parents are inadequate or hurtful. Maintaining narratives in which their own deficiencies were the cause of their parents' hurtfulness or neglectful allows them to hold on to relationships that insure their survival. Other children cling to myths of a parents' "greatness" to maintain idealizing ties during times when their need for guidance and protection is particularly strong as in periods of societal conflict or during natural disasters. Analysts often report that their patients' discoveries about their parents' inadequacies were turning points in their healing relationships.

Those of us who have treated couples may be especially aware that at the time when people chose their spouses, they seem not to have known about the very aspects of their future partner's personality that they later identify as problematic for the relationship. Knowing these things might well have stopped the relationship from proceeding. The reasons for not knowing problematic aspects of a prospective spouse are too numerous to list. Some cannot bear knowing that their future spouses resembled a hated relative, or that they embody aspects of themselves they find shameful. Others simply believe it was time to get married and knowing would have made marriage impossible. The focus on couples' therapy is often on discovering if the relationship can thrive when what was once disavowed becomes known. See Chapter 7 on the ways we view the need to know and the need not to know in couples therapy.

The Need Not to Know We

If we-connectedness is indispensable for one's development of a sense of self, it makes sense that knowing anything that diminishes these bonds jeopardizes one's psychological survival. The need not to know negative aspects of a we-connection may lead us to accept falsehoods about the superiority of our group and the inferiority of others. In Chapter 8 we examine how the need to know and not know organizes communities.

The Need Not to Know World

In these troubled times, many of our patients have told us that they simply cannot bear knowing about the horrendous wars that are being waged in the world, the slow destruction of our planet caused by human-generated climate change, and the shameful behavior of political leaders. Some have limited their exposure to the news and some have even forbidden guests at social gatherings from mentioning politics. Much as we too would like to copy such ostrich-like avoidance, we feel that it is valuable to keep ourselves open to talking with patients about world events. We have often found that the very world situations about which patients wish not to know have deep meanings in their own lives. (We devote Chapter 10 to an exploration of our embodied relational knowing needs in the context of the world.)

Psychoanalytic Healing and the Need Not to Know

We do not believe that every instance of not knowing can be eliminated by even the most thoroughgoing analytic treatment. There always seem to be fresh aspects of our lives and those of our patients that we need not to know. However, we have experienced the diminution of this need as trust develops between the analytic partners. We suspect that trust is more likely to deepen when our empathy is infused with our awareness that we meet our patients, and they meet us as what we call "foreign bodies" (see Chapter 1). That is, when we allow ourselves to become aware of the limits of our empathic capacity and recognize that humans are all unknowable to some extent in their uniqueness, the therapeutic relationship seems to open to what are new opportunities for healing.

References

Atwood, G. E. & Stolorow, R. D. (1980). Psychoanalytic Concepts and the Representational World. *Psychoanal. Contemp. Thought*, 3: 267–290.

Atwood, G. E. & Stolorow, R. D. (1981). Experience and Conduct. *Contemporary Psychoanalysis*, 17: 197–208.

Beebe, B. & Lachmann, F. (2014). *The Origin of Attachment: Infant Research and Adult Treatment.* London and New York: Routledge Taylor & Francis Group.

BOK, S. (1983), The Limits of Confidentiality. Hastings Center Report, 13: 24–31.

Bromberg, P. M. (2011). *The Shadow of the Tsunami and the Growth of the Relational Mind.* London and New York: Routledge Taylor & Francis Group.

Brothers, D. (2008). *Toward a Psychology of Uncertainty – Trauma-Centered Psychoanalysis.* London and New York: The Analytic Press Taylor & Francis Group.

Brothers, D. (2014). Traumatic Attachments: Intergenerational Trauma, Dissociation and the Analytic Relationship. *International Journal of Psychoanalytic Self Psychology*, 9: 1, 3–15.

Brothers, D. & Sletvold, J. (2022). Talking Bodies: A New Vision of Psychoanalysis. Psychoanalytic Inquiry. 42:4, 289–302. DOI: 10.1080/07351690.2022.2059292

Brothers, D. & Sletvold, J. (2023). *A New Vision of Psychoanalytic Theory, Practice and Supervision: TALKING BODIES.* London and New York: Routledge Taylor & Francis Group.

Frie, R. (2017). *Not in My Family: German Memory and Responsibility After the Holocaust.* Oxford, U.K Oxford University Press.

Freud, S. (1905 [1904]). *On Psychotherapy*. The Standard Edition of the Complete Psychological Works of Sigmund Freud. 7: 255–268.

Sletvold, J. (2014). *The Embodied Mind – From Freud and Reich to Relationality.* London and New York: Routledge Taylor & Francis Group.

Spitz, R. A. (1957). *No and Yes. On the Genesis of Human Communication*. Unknown Edition.

Spitz, R. A. (1965). *The First Year of life: A psychoanalytic Study of Normal Development of Object Relations.* New York: International Universities Press. Dimensons.

Stern, D. B. (2010). *Partners in Thought – Working with Unformulated Experience, Dissociation, and Enactment.* London and New York: Routledge Taylor & Francis Group.

Stolorow, R. D. (2006). Autobiographical and Theoretical Reflections on the "Ontological Unconscious". *Contemporary Psychoanalysis*, 42: 233–241.

Winnicott, D. W. (1965). *The Maturational Process and the Facilitating Environment: Studies in the Theory of Emotional Development*. London: Hogarth Press. 64: 37–55.

Ulman, R. B. & Brothers, D. (1988). *The Shattered Self – A Psychoanalytic Study of Trauma.* Hillsdale, NJ and London: The Analytic Press.

Zerbe, K. (2019). The Secret Life of Secrets: Deleterious Psychosomatic Effects on Patients and Analysts. *Journal of the American Psychoanalytic Association*, 67: 185–214.

Zerbe, K. (2025). *Secrets in Psychotherapy: Stories that Inform Clinical Work*. New York; Routledge. ISBN: 9781003471578

3 Knowing Dreams

In our dreams, the past, and even the future, may enter a strange, mysterious present. People long dead may mingle with the living. Events seemingly forgotten may recur with fresh intensity. What occurs in our nighttime travels can seem more vividly real—even more terrifyingly so—than what we experience during our waking hours. But what stands out most compellingly for us as we write this book is that some dreams form a bridge between our need to know (and be known) and our need not to know (and not to be known). It is common, for example, that what patients may have needed not to know when they went to sleep, may become available for them to know when they reflect on their dreams after they wake up—especially when they tell the dreams to their analysts.

In his masterpiece, *The Interpretation of Dreams*, hailed for its groundbreaking theory of unconscious processes, Freud (1913) identified the manifest content of the dream as the narrative remembered by the dreamer while the latent content contained its unconscious meaning. We would say a dream's meaning is better understood as being prereflectively unconscious (Atwood and Stolorow, 1980, 1981) insofar as its meaning often becomes available to consciousness in analytic dialogues. We prefer to think of the latent content in terms of the need not to know insofar as we have found that the strength and duration of this need depends on the context in which the dream is remembered and told as well as the timing of the dream's emergence.

It is common to find that aspects of a dream have been disguised. For example, a person who appears in a dream may not be the one the dreamer has had strong feelings about. The dreamer prefers not to know who the dream person stands for. We would never consider calling the dreamer a liar for this subterfuge. We might instead imagine that the dreamer has gone to great lengths not to know the dream's meaning. But, as we shall see in Chapter 10, when the need not to know collides with the need to know about world events, lies are often told.

Since 1913, the year in which "The Interpretation of Dreams" was published, a plethora of theories of dreaming have emerged. In recent years,

DOI: 10.4324/9781003487883-4

neuroscientists and cognitive researchers have discovered how brains behave during sleep. Who has not heard of REM, rapid eye movement periods during sleep? Rahul Jandial (2024), a neuroscientist and brain surgeon, asserts that the dreaming brain is as active as the waking brain and that the amount of energy in the emotional and visual centers of the brain during dreaming can exceed that of the waking brain. In his 2024 book, "This Is Why You Dream," Jandial, reviews some of the theories supporting the idea that dreams are not random and probably have had evolutionary value. They include the ideas that dreams serve the purpose of threat rehearsal, help us metabolize anxiety-provoking emotions, function as a means of testing interpersonal situations, and keep the neural networks functioning during sleep. No theory, he contends, has emerged as the single reason humans dream and suggests that all are valid to some degree.

We will not review the many different ways in which psychoanalysts have understood dreaming but recommend an issue of Psychoanalytic Dialogues (1999) co-edited by Lewis Aron and James Fosshage and articles by Fosshage (2007, 2024) if you wish to learn more about these ideas.

Our intention in what follow is by no means to develop a new theory of dreams. It may be that all dreams may be understood in terms of the need to know and the need not to know. However, in what follows we focus on those dreams in which the intersection between the different aspects of embodied relational knowing is particularly notable. Doris offers one of her dreams as an example:

> During a period of intense grief over my father's death, I (Doris) had a dream, a snippet of which I recall as follows: I am dancing with my father at a party of some sort, and I jokingly say to him, "You dance pretty well for a dead guy."

On waking, I suddenly realized that, until that moment, I had needed not to know that my father had died. Before the dream I had often imagined that he was nearby when the gait of a far-off stranger resembled his, or a laugh had the same hearty peal. My dream seems to have told me that I had finally accepted that my father was dead. In days following this dream the heaviness of my sorrow lessened (although I continued to miss him sorely, as I do to this day). Instead of brooding over his last days of suffering, I could remember the happy times we shared.

What made me able to accept the reality of my father's death when I did? I cannot say for sure, but I imagine that some friends or relatives had contacted me in my grief in a way allowed me to face life without my father.

When I told this dream to members of a supervision/study group (see Chapter 9), one of the members, Dr. Teodor Negulescu (we call him Teo), remembered a dream he had the day after his mother died. Here is the write-up of the dream Teo kindly sent to us:

> *I am in the entrance hall to the first place where I ever lived—a communist grey bloc of flats. I am with my father and my brother and there is a sort of bulletin board on the wall, with a mirror. I look in the mirror and I see my mother standing behind me. I turn to her, and she says, "My key is not working anymore". I talk back to her in a parental tone: "Let's see what's going on, I'm going to fix this right now". I put the key in the door, and I suddenly realize I am dreaming. I wake up.*

Interpreting his own dream, Teo wrote: *"I so wanted to lose contact with the reality of her being gone." Yet, as Teo later explained, he had needed to "stay in the reality" of what was happening during the time his mother was dying. He had greatly supported his father and brother by "staying resolutely adult." He noted that much as he had determined not even to dream that his mother was still alive, he had a forbidden but strong wish to do so.*

Teo's dream is the inverse of Doris's. Whereas Doris's dream seemed to indicate her readiness to know the reality of her father's death, Teo's dream indicated his wish not to know his mother's death was real. Perhaps he needed more time to process his painful loss. Nevertheless, these dreams illustrate how dreaming can serve either to help our need to know or not to know the reality of some emotionally powerful event such as the death of a loved one.

After we wrote this part of the chapter, Jon's mother also appeared in one of his dreams. Here is how he remembers it:

> *I'm presenting a paper at a conference that is being held near where a dear childhood friend lives. I decide to visit him. After saying goodbye to him, I take a train to the home where I'm living with my mother. When I see her, I say to myself, "It's okay to live with one's mother when one is a very young man."*

As we discussed his dream, Jon remembered that before going to sleep, he had been thinking about how he felt about his mother at the time of her death and in the present. What he suddenly realized as he thought about the dream's ending was that he longed to be young again. As a young man he could be taken care of instead of being the one who provides care for others. Jon's dream had followed a particularly difficult day of sessions with patients who had implored him to relieve their emotional pain. As we talked about his dream, Jon mentioned that, characteristically, he had not wanted to know his feeling of being overwhelmed by the burdens he carries.

It is not surprising that the interpretation of dreams has become a hallmark of psychoanalytic therapy. In what follows, we provide examples of dreams that demonstrate how they bridge needing to know and needing not to know. Our examination of the dreams that follow is somewhat abbreviated and hardly exhaust all of the possible meanings they held for the dreamer and the analyst.

Dreams That Mark the Healing Process

Although neither the patient nor the analyst ever fully knows how the analysis is changing a patient's life, a dream may allow them to better understand the healing process. The following dream is illustrative:

Mel, a talented writer, was the youngest child in a family of high achievers. We suspect that his obvious intellectual gifts had aroused intense competition and envy from his siblings, a reason perhaps that he had always stayed out of the limelight. He frequently downplayed his own accomplishments and even failed to inform his analyst when a book he had been writing for many years was accepted for publication by a noted publishing house. After a session in which the analyst suggested that his painful experiences with his siblings might have contributed to his delay in informing the analyst of the book's publication, Mel had the following dream:

> *I am sitting in the audience at an award ceremony when I think I might have heard my name called to receive an award. Not sure that I had heard correctly, I stayed seated. When my name was called again, even louder this time, I realized that I would receive an award. I stumbled as I climbed the steps of the stage, but I was supported by the person holding an enormous trophy that had my name inscribed on it.*

After telling the dream, Mel said that he had never allowed himself to think he might be given a literary award, but that nothing would mean more to him than to have his work recognized by other writers. We imagine that Mel's need not to be known for his talent as a writer and for all his other accomplishments and attributes had contributed to his survival in a highly competitive family. Although he had accepted his position as "the ordinary child" to gain some sense of certainty that his emotional needs might be met, his need for recognition had not been extinguished. It was only after his analyst had helped him to understand what had made it necessary to hide his achievements and had affirmed his need for recognition that he was able imagine being recognized for his unique talents.

Another dream that revealed more about an analytic relationship was told by Molly, the patient Doris describes in Chapter 4, "Knowing Power." Molly reported the following dream s few months after her late boyfriend, Gene, had died:

> *I'm shopping for a dress with Gene in a high-end store. He insists that I buy a dress that I think is wrong for me. I wear the dress to a restaurant and feel embarrassed and uncomfortable.*

Discussing the dream, Molly remembered that her father bought her a watch when she graduated high school that she described as "a cheap, ugly thing that would have been better suited for a boy." For the first time, she connected her boyfriend with her father. "Neither man had a clue about who I am, and neither man really cared about pleasing me" she said. We talked about her faulty efforts to wrest power from both men and others in her life, which we both felt held enormous significance for her. We discuss the power dynamics in the analytic relationship between Molly and Doris in Chapter 4.

Dreams Anticipating Change

Sometimes a dream image seems to shout its message that a patient is ready to change through images that are blatantly obvious. Such was the case with Mara. Although Mara faced a work-related challenge that was almost identical to several she had faced in the past, she had needed not to know about the role she played in the situation. Once again, Mara had spoken harshly to an employee who subsequently complained about her to her superiors. Mara had insisted that her criticism had been justified and that the employee was another overly sensitive "bad apple." After the situation had been explored in great depth in several sessions, Mara had begun to glimpse how she might have provoked the repetition. She then had the following dream.

> *A huge owl enters through an open window in my bedroom and appears to be flying directly toward a wall of mirrors. Suddenly it veers and escapes through an opening in a wall.*

Asked to say what she imagined the dream meant, Mara said, "Owls are supposed to be wise. I think the dream is about knowing something that I didn't know I was smart enough to know." Then Mara said, I have gotten through many tough times in my life, and I've done so through confrontations—like if the owl had crashed into the mirror. Maybe I can find another way through these situations.

In fact, Mara had been subjected to relentless criticism by both parents. But turning the tables and experiencing herself as the hurtful criticizer had almost cost her a job and her reputation. The obvious image of the owl as the knower, seems to have told Mara that she needed to know how she contributed to her work problems. She was ready to find another way.

A dream also signaled that change was now possible for Gloria, an attractive and well-educated middle-aged woman, who was quite overweight. She had entered therapy with Doris by saying that she needed help with her "gluttony." "I just can't discipline myself to stay on a diet," she complained. During the analysis, she remembered that she had first put on weight at age 14, soon after her father had touched her breast and genitals. Because he had not attempted intercourse, she had not considered his molestation to constitute sexual abuse. It slowly became clear to her that her life-long avoidance of sexual relationships was not because "no man wants to have sex with a fat girl," but because she could not bear a repetition of the disappointment she had felt when her father had molested her.

After trying one of the new weight-reduction medications and losing some weight, she reported the following dream.

> *I'm at a resort with Jason Maroma, a gorgeous actor. We cannot find a private room to be alone together. I am wearing only my bra and panties, but Jason seems to want to have sex with me despite my bulges. I am overcome with embarrassment, but we decide that we will find some way to be together.*

As we talked about the dream over the next several sessions. Gloria again mentioned that her weight gain had begun after her father had molested her. "I now understand that I would not have bulges today if it hadn't happened," she said. Gloria then suddenly realized that she had needed not to know that her father, whom she had greatly idealized, had disappointed her even before the molestation. Although he had been considered a model of ethical behavior in their community, her mother had revealed that he had frequently been unfaithful in the marriage. Gloria now understood that the padding of fat she had accumulated had helped her to avoid knowing painful truths: she was attractive to men and that it was her father, not her, whose behavior was morally reprehensible. The dream of being attractive to a man she found so desirable also allowed her to know that she was ready to find a relationship in which sexual desire was mutually shared.

We offer still another dream heralding change in a patient whose romantic relationships had always ended in painful rejections. Wendy, an attractive and accomplished woman of 45, had spent much of her time in her weekly sessions bemoaning the fact that Bob, the man she had recently fallen in love with, refused to give up his other sexual partners. She felt that the only way to keep him connected to her was to accept his unwillingness to be a faithful partner.

Wendy had grown up in a household where her father's illness had dominated the family's lives. Her mother seemed more devoted to attending to his needs than to Wendy and her brother, Wendy's mother seems to have modeled the role of the self-sacrificing woman who served the man's need above all else.

Although Wendy had dated many men, she had never felt worthy of their admiration or even respect. As the attention in analysis focused on the possibility that her poor sense of self was connected to her inability to feel that her mother wished to know her and care for her, she had begun to imagine finding a truly reciprocal relationship. During this period in her analysis, she had the following dream:

> *Bob is in a room with many women who want to have sex with him. When I look at him, I see that he is huge—about twice my size. I say to myself. "I can't be with a man that big."*

Discussing the dream. Wendy realized that although she had allowed Bob to hold all the power in the relationship, she didn't like it. "Maybe," she said for the first time, "I could live without him." Her belief that the only way to have a man was to be like her mother was finally under question. We suspect that feeling connected to her analyst as a caring maternal figure had enabled her to feel that change was possible.

Anxiety Dreams

According to Jandial (2024) dreams have maintained a remarkable consistency over the span of human history and across societies. In a research study the dreams of American, Japanese and German students revealed remarkable similarity. Among the most frequent dreams are those that involved falling, trying again and again to do something, and those about school, teachers, and studying,

We have been told many dreams by different patients over the years that are typically understood as "anxiety dreams." These include the dreamer's being late for an important event such as a meeting or an examination, having failed to measure up to some school or professional requirement, being naked in public, and being chased. We have found that when a dream of this sort involves the intersection of the need to know and the need not to know, the meanings may be very specific to the dreamer. Here is an example:

Beth, a senior in high school, had been locked in a continual struggle with her controlling parents. They fought over the sports she should play, the colleges should she apply to, the friends that could be invited home, even the boys she could date.

When Beth told her analyst a dream in which she is informed during her graduation ceremony that she cannot graduate because she lacks two credits to meet the school requirement, the initial discussion focused on her anxiety. " 'I'm very anxious about keeping up my grades during this last semester before I graduate," she said." She explained that she very much wanted to graduate with honors in math and science. However, as the session progressed, Beth seemed to become increasingly sad. Abandoning her usual fast-paced, almost frantic way of talking, she spoke in quiet monotone. Finally, she said, "I'm afraid to be accepted into college." I don't want to go away from home." Then she said, "What am I saying? Of course, I want to get as far away from my parents as possible."

As we explored her surprising and contradictory reactions, the meaning of her dream became clearer. Failing to have the credits needed for graduation meant that she could stay home. Despite their involvement in every aspect of her life, her parents had failed to meet Beth's needs for their recognition of unique qualities. They had simply wanted to enjoy her accomplishments. Beth was not prepared to face college life without these missed experiences. Her dream seemed to reveal what she needed not to know: that she longed to stay home to finally have what she valued in herself recognized by her parents.

Another common dream that seems to have specific meanings for the dreamer involves being chased. A good example is the one we offer below:

Effie, a successful 54-year-old corporate executive, had been chased over and over again in her childhood dreams by a variety of "bad guys" including villains in scary movies she had seen. One of the reasons she had sought analysis was her fear of dying in some dreadful accident or natural disaster. After the first few months, little mention was made of her fear until it was revived when a colleague was killed in a plane crash. She then had the following dream:

> *I am walking alone down the road where I live when the streetlights go out and I hear footsteps behind me. I turn to look but I see no one. I'm terrified as the sound of the footsteps gets louder and louder. I wake up with a pounding heart.*

When the meaning of her dream was explored, Effie's fear of death seemed obvious. "Death, "she said, "has always been chasing me." She then wondered if her childhood dreams of being chased had begun after the death of her beloved grandmother. However, the tragic loss of her colleagues in a plane crash appears not to have been the only impetus for her dream. What she had needed not to know and consequently had not mentioned in her analytic sessions was that she had been suffering from symptoms suggestive of Parkinson's disease. It is still uncertain if she is suffering from this disease, but she was grateful that the dream provided her with the chance to share her fear with her analyst.

Analysts' and Patients' Dreams of One Another

Perhaps the most dramatic ways in which relational knowing needs of patient and analyst are illuminated in dreams involves those in which a patient dreams about the analyst or the analyst dreams about a patient. One of Doris' dreams is particularly revealing in this respect.

> *I'm in a park near where i used to live with my two young children. They are busily playing when a little girl appears. I think, "Oh, yes, I have three children. How could I have forgotten?"*

The dream was very unsettling for me, and I wondered if the child might have represented an aspect of myself. Even if I understood how this could be true, I suspected that the deeper dream message was eluding me. It was only when my patient, Jenny, appeared for her session that I recalled that little girl in the dream looked just as Jenny might have looked as a young child. I had occasionally felt some slight stirrings of maternal feeling for her, but this feeling rarely entered my thoughts about our work.

Jenny's reasons for entering analysis had always been vague. She had a decent job, a reasonably happy marriage, and her two children appeared to be thriving. Although her parents were divorced, her descriptions of her childhood were filled with stories of happy celebrations and lovely vacations. Nevertheless, she appeared for her sessions on time and filled them with accounts of slight disruptions in her relationships with friends and minor upsets with her husband and children. I (Doris) had suspected that Jenny had needed more from her analysis than what she gave as her oft repeated reason: "I want to learn all I can about myself." My dream helped me find out what it was that she needed.

In the session that followed I asked Jenny to tell me more about her mother. She began by telling me how accomplished her mother was as a pianist, how devoted she was to her church and how she had tirelessly volunteered in community projects. Then she said in a very quiet voice, "it was very different when she was drinking." In answer to my questions, Jenny explained that her mother's alcoholism had resulted in her being extremely neglectful. She often slept so late in the mornings that Jenny had to prepare her own breakfast and school lunch. She sometimes started drinking soon after Jenny returned from school. Jenny wept as she spoke of envying other children who could turn to their mothers for comfort in times of trouble.

Much changed after her mother sought psychological help and began to attend AA meetings. Jenny confessed that in telling new friends about her mother she would omit any mention of her drinking. "I was even ashamed to let you know about it," she said.

Needless to say, the dream and the sessions that followed greatly changed our relationship as Jenny spoke openly about her feeling that I could be the mother she would not have been ashamed of.

Why, Doris wondered, had she needed not to know that the dream was about Jenny? After much reflection, she realized that the third child in the dream may have represented her own mother, whose own unmet needs for mothering had greatly affected Doris' life.

A dream by one of Doris's patients about her was similarly meaningful.

Perhaps the earliest and most significant event in Jean's young life was the death of her mother when Jean was only four years old. Her mother's long illness probably began shortly after the birth of Jean's younger brother when Jean was two. Jean was left in the care of a couple who were rigid in their demands and harshly punitive in response to any acts of childish mischief. Since Jean's father's self-centeredness was intensified by his loss of his wife, it was little wonder that Jean felt that she had been orphaned by her mother's death.

Jean's first marriage to a caring and accomplished man ended tragically when he died after a devastating illness. After several years of grieving, Jean fell in love with Dan, whose intense sexual attraction for her felt irresistible. Jean realized that Dan was somewhat withholding and self-involved. Yet, after much hesitation and ambivalence, Jean accepted his marriage proposal.

Jean reported the following snippet of a dream a few months after their marriage.

> *Dan is sitting in a café with you (Doris) and his eyes are glittering with lust. You seem to be naked but when I try to look at your naked breasts, I see that your body is covered by a sort of thin meshy material that obscures your nipples. I feel disappointed that I can't see them.*

Our discussion of Jean's dream confirmed my concern that Dan was very much like her father (she knew that he had many sexual affairs while married to Jean's mother). It also seemed to confirm her much disguised longing for me as a maternal figure who would offer her the warmth and nurturing that she had always craved.

Although I had sensed Jean's longing for me as the mother she had lost, she had previously spurned any suggestion that she might hope to recapture with me her missed experiences of being mothered. Hearing the dream, I realized that I had protected myself (the covered nipples?) against feeling hurt by her denials by avoiding mentioning my concern about her marriage to Dan.

We began our exploration of the dream by talking about Jean's possible sexual desire for me. It soon became clear that sexual feelings were far safer for her to acknowledge than her longings for maternal care. What if, like her mother and first husband, I too might die or otherwise leave her? In discussing the dream, Jean also realized that she wanted my help in confronting Dan's potential infidelity and tendency to withdraw emotionally. Although I never voiced this, I imagined that this was just what a mother might have offered in such matters.

It seems probable that Jean told her dream to me in the hope that I would better understand the complex nature of her feelings for me. It also greatly helped me understand my feelings for her.

Summary

We hope that by viewing dreams as the bridging of needing to know and not to know, we provide a new way to treasure the gift of dreams, those precious jewels of psychoanalytic practice.

References

Aron, L. & Fosshage, J. (1999). The Interpretation of Dreams: A Centennial Celebration. *Psychoanalytic Dialogues*, 9(6): 721–724.

Atwood, G. E. & Stolorow, R. D. (1980). Psychoanalytic Concepts and the Representational World. *Psychoanal. Contemp. Thought*, 3: 267–290.

Atwood, G. E. & Stolorow, R. D. (1981). Experience and Conduct. *Contemporary Psychoanalysis*, 17: 197–208.

Fosshage, J. (2007). The Organizing Function of Dreams: Pivotal Issues in Understanding and Working with Dreams. *International Journal of Psychoanalysis*, 16: 213–221.
Fosshage, J. (2024). Is Dreaming Thinking? Pivotal Issues in Understanding and Working with Dreams. *Psychoanalytic Inquiry*, 44: 816–826.
Freud, S. (1913). *The Interpretation of Dreams*. Trans. A. A. Brill. Macmillan. (Original work published 1900).
Jandial, R. (2024). *This Is Why You Dream*. London: Penguin Random House, UK.

4 Knowing Power

We could not imagine exploring the relationship between embodied relational knowing and power in the analytic setting without referring to Michel Foucault (Foucault & Gordon, 1980) since these intertwined concepts represent a central theme in his work. Believing that his ideas deepen our understanding of analytic relationships, we refer to his work extensively in this chapter and refer to him in several others. We are well aware that his ideas have been criticized for reflecting his radical views on sexuality and politics. Among these are his sanctioning of all forms of consensual sex, including pedophilia. However, as Silverman (2003) and Eribon (1991) point out, when he was confronted with the implications of his radical views, he often moderated them and even abandoned some. And, it goes without saying that we believe that what he has contributed is not diminished by the controversy that surrounds him.

For Foucault, power is so intimately connected to knowledge that he coined the term, "power-knowledge." By putting the words, "power" and "knowledge" together, Foucault attempted to demonstrate that power is always based on knowledge and that its influence is found everywhere in our lives and in our society. As Forrester (2017, p. 216) points out, Foucault attacked the enlightenment battle of knowledge over ignorance with its belief that scientific knowledge is opposed to power and that it will win out over the forces of oppression. Contradicting this view, Foucault showed that knowledge can never be innocent of its origins and effects.

Foucault notes that power and knowledge come to be joined in discourse. We find that the linkage of power and knowledge in the analytic exchange does not necessarily require the use of words. Consider his statement:

> All men by nature desire to know; the proof of this is caused by sensations, forever apart from their usefulness, we enjoy them for themselves.
>
> (Foucault, 1977, p. 5)

To the extent that Foucault asserts that power-knowledge involves pleasure and sensations, it seems clear that it is an embodied phenomenon for him.

DOI: 10.4324/9781003487883-5

Moreover, he even asserts that the way power operates societally is exercised on bodies. For example, he writes:

> What I want to show is how power relations can materially penetrate the body in depth, without depending on the subjects' own representations. If power takes hold on the body, this isn't through it's having to be interiorized in people's consciousness.
>
> (Foucault, 1977, p. 186)

Foucault explains that what he calls "the circuit of bio-power" or "somatic-power," acts as the formative matrix of sexuality and operates within the historical and cultural milieu in which we live. While we are also interested in the ways in which power and knowledge involve sexuality as a societal phenomenon (see Chapter 5) we are more concerned with the effects of the link between power and knowing in the workings of every analytic encounter.

Rather than viewing power in binaries such as powerful and weak, or dominant and submissive, or doer and done to, we see power, especially as it manifests in therapeutic relationships as a constantly shifting phenomenon that must be thought of in terms of degree. It is very much a question of "more or less." As Foucault (1977) puts it,

> Power is exercised rather than possessed, and it is sometimes employed by those who are dominated. We view the exercise of power as a relational phenomenon, not as something that exists solely within the individual.
>
> (Foucault, 1977, pp. 26–27)

For us, the shifts in power to which Foucault refers are very closely connected to shifts in our embodied relational knowing needs. Our own and our patients' needs not to know cognitively what we may know on a bodily level depends on what power relations are being enacted in an analytic dialogue. When memories of painful imbalances of power are revived by what is happening between patient and analyst, the need not to know may intensify.

Douglas Vakoch (1998, p. 339), referring to Foucault, notes that the analyst can use the familiar space of the consulting room to exert a subtle yet constraining power over the patient. We agree that the activities that organize the analytic setting play a large role in analytic power relations. Analysts may be perceived as powerful insofar as they engage in such quotidian practices as setting the analytic session times, controlling the fee arrangements, determining the vacation breaks, etc. While many writers have referred to the asymmetry of the analytic relationships in terms of the analyst's power, the choices that patients make within these arrangements may affect the power relations as well. For example, patients may choose to show up for sessions or not, to come on time or not, to pay the fee on time or not, and, of course, patients may end the therapeutic relationship at any time.

But more importantly, analysts and patients tend to exert power to the extent that both control what is permissible for the other to know. Although we are familiar with the idea that analysts tend to restrict their verbal self-disclosures, (especially among more traditionally Freudian analysts) patients also continually choose what they say about themselves and how fully they do so (see Chapter 2). This is especially true with respect to their feelings about their analysts. Patients may also be experienced as powerful to the extent that they induce their analysts to make themselves known.

The Power of Confession

Power and embodied relational knowing are strongly linked in the analytic situation when considered in terms of the ways in which Foucault understands "confession." Although we tend to associate confession with religion, particularly the Catholic religion, Foucault famously associated it with sexuality. Noting that Western societies have developed "scientia sexualis" (scientific sexuality) rather than "ars sexualis" (erotic art), he asserts that ours is

> the only civilization to have developed over the centuries procedures for telling the truth of sex which are geared to a form of knowledge-power strictly opposed to the art of initiations and masterful secret: I have in mind the confession.
>
> (Foucault, 1976, p. 58)

He has suggested that confessions, especially about sexuality, are a feature of most intimate relationships.

Free association, the guiding principle of early Freudian practice, involved the idea that patients must disclose their thoughts, feelings, fantasies, wishes, dreams, and particularly those that were sexual, to their analysts—even if they violated societal expectations. We assume that many patients experienced such disclosures as confessions. But just as confessing one's "sins" to a priest may be relieving so these confessions to one's analyst may prove immensely gratifying. In Foucault's (1976, p. 82) words: "The one who confesses is, conversely, unburdened of his wrongs, liberated."

However, since a confession is only worthwhile if it heard by another person (or religious entity), and patients are not expected to hear their analysts' confessions, the power dynamics of the analytic situation may be experienced as greatly skewed toward the analysts. Analysts are granted the privilege of knowing the darkest, most shameful aspects of their patients' lives while they rarely reciprocate this level of knowing with their patients.

Clearly confessing and hearing confessions are not merely cognitive exchanges. They are often intensely feeling-laden for both the person who confesses and the person hearing the confession. As Foucault suggests, even the impulse to confess may be related to changes in ourselves that have been produced by the power dynamic of the analytic relationship.

Some patients confess in order to feel greater intimacy with their analysts, a means of escaping crippling loneliness. For others, it brings relief from the burden of keeping dark secrets hidden. For still others it may seem like the only way to keep the analyst's attention—the more gut-wrenching the confession the more likely it seems that the analyst is bound to them.

Analysts also make confessions, often with their bodies. Without uttering a word, they may confess their liking, dislike, irritation, disgust or their sexual desire for their patients by subtle changes in their bodies. While patients may perceive these feelings, which may not even be conscious for the analyst, they may feel prohibited from knowing them cognitively for fear of alienating them. The power wielded by analysts may be very great to the extent that patients are constrained by their need for the analysts' help.

When the word, "power," appears in psychoanalytic contexts it has usually connoted some negative experience. We often think of power, as Jessica Benjamin (1988, 2004) has suggested, in terms of doer and done to. However, power may also be understood more broadly as simply having the ability to do something or having the ability to influence others. Political scientists have taught us that power does not necessarily require force or threat but may involve much subtler means.

We have the idea that just by acting as analysts--or patients for that matter, we are exerting power. In one of Joseph Lichtenberg's (2024) last papers, he also described the ubiquitous nature of power in the therapeutic relationship. He writes:

> We propose that a common theme that animates all motivational activity is the sense of power. Power refers to the experience of can-do, of being a doer doing. Maintaining a sense of power, when conceptualized as the primary motivational goal of daily life, moves psychoanalytic theory from the abstract to the personal. The main focus in therapy, thus, is moved from past experiences to the greater significance of the present moment.
>
> (Lichtenberg, 2024, p. 791)

As we attempt to show in our clinical illustrations, the more we-connectedness develops between the analytic partners, the more both tend to feel powerful. Power then is not perceived as having been used to diminish the other person, but, rather, is shared. We find that a sense of increased power—often experienced as having greater agency and freedom to choose—is the strongest indicator that healing has occurred for both patient and analyst.

Power and Envy

Not knowing on a cognitive level what we know on a bodily level about power may allow us to avoid experiencing tension with patients whom we perceive as having higher or lower status, greater or lesser professional standing, more or less wealth, beauty, grace, talent, and so on, than we do.

This brings us to a consideration of the relationship between power and envy. Louis Sass (forthcoming) has studied envy among the Purépecha Mexicans, who, in contrast to most members of contemporary Western societies, consider envy to be a central aspect of their lives. According to Sass, Helmut Schoeck (1966/1969) attributes the fact that envy has largely been ignored by social scientists since the beginning of the 20th century to a kind of societal repression. In line with his idea, it is interesting to consider that although most relational analysts are familiar with Freud's account of "penis envy" and Melanie Kein's idea that the roots of envy are to be found in infancy, they usually mention envy only in relation to severe psychological disorders.

When viewed through the lens of embodied relational knowing, envy seems mainly to reside in the realm of the need not to know. We suspect that a common reason not to know that we envy a powerful other is that knowing often leads to shame; the very experience of envying another's power is evidence of our experience of shameful inferiority. But even the person who is envied as powerful may feel shame. In many cultures, the idea of glorying in one's superiority is strongly frowned upon.

We have identified what we believe to be a common means of avoiding the feeling of envy; It involves attempts to "become" the person who is envied. Patients who experience themselves as like their analysts by imitating their manner of speaking, dressing, etc. may, to some extent, be avoiding envious feelings. The experience tends to level the perceived power imbalances in the relationship.

A patient Doris described in our 2023 book who seemed to believe that her thoughts and feelings were shared by Doris, may well have needed to avoid experiences of envy (Brothers & Sletvold, 2023, pp. 31–32). As the relationship developed, the patient remembered instances in which her mother (whom she experienced as intensely envious) had often presented herself as an age-mate rather than a guiding protective figure for the patient. We now wonder if by following her mother's example she too could avoid feeling envy.

Those who are envied may seem to be unaware of the power they hold and the envy they elicit. An exceptionally beautiful patient of Jon's, for example, could not understand why so many women friends acted in hurtful, albeit disguised, ways toward her. When Jon examined each instance of "meanness" on the part of a friend, the patient was shocked by her realization that the hurtful act was motivated by envy.

The tendency to act in destructive ways toward those who are envied is very common. As Sass notes,

> Only with envy does aggression take aim at the excellent or the good precisely *because* of its excellence or its goodness—whether this be possessions, relationships, or inherent attributes of the envied other. The envier's desire, presumably, is less to acquire something good than to diminish or destroy the envied one.

While we doubt that envy always involves destructive wishes, those of us who have received negative reviews by patients may have been victims of envious reprisal. We suggest that when some patients need not to know that they envy the analyst's power to heal, their desire to diminish the analyst's power may lead to hate in the relationship (see Chapter 5). We believe that this is just as likely to result when analysts need not to know that they envy their patients.

Even if, as we are suggesting, both patients and analysts tend to need not to know their envy of the power held by the other, knowing may nevertheless register on a bodily level. It is also interesting to consider how our bodily appearance affects perceptions of power and envy. A man who had been terribly bullied in his family, exclaimed on first seeing Doris after the initial phone contact. "Oh, you're so little!" Although, at first, both Doris and this patient, believed that he was unhappy to be in analysis with a woman whose short stature suggested weakness, they later discovered how relieved he was to find that Doris seemed to lack physical strength. Indeed, he eventually admitted his envy of the fact, that as a woman, she seemed to have no need to be tall and muscular. This patient had spent much of his time weightlifting at a gym to make himself look immune to repetitions of physical bullying.

We now offer some clinical examples to illustrate our ideas about power, envy and embodied relational knowing.

Molly and Doris

In the first months of my analytic relationship with Molly, a woman of 85 who needed two canes to walk because of a serious movement disorder, I (Doris) could not utter a sentence that she would not correct. I imagined that if I said, "it's sunny out today," Molly would have said, "Don't you see the clouds?" When I commented on her needing to correct me, she predictably answered. "No, not all the time."

Despite the relative insignificance of her criticisms, some of which seemed remarkably trivial to me, I experienced Molly as quite powerful. I felt compelled to learn how to address her in ways that would not need correcting. I also felt disempowered by my inability to even imagine what was going on between us. Molly seemed to like me, and I enjoyed her wit and playfulness, but her continual quibbling about the accuracy of my comments unnerved me.

Molly had come to see me because of her disappointment in her long-time companion, Gene, a 90-year-old man with whom she had established a sexual relationship years earlier, while his wife was still alive. After, his wife died, Gene had moved into Molly's apartment but had not shared equally in the expenses. Nor had he agreed to provide for her in his will. Instead, he often gave a great deal of money to his already well-off sons, both of whom regarded Molly with contempt as "the mistress."

Whenever I attempted to understand her relationship with Gene in greater depth, Molly would become even more critical of how I spoke. I assumed that most of her corrections were intended to protect Gene from anything that sounded like criticism of him on my part. When, for example, I told her that she seemed hurt when she realized that Gene had not provided for her in his will, she said "Well, he did say that somehow I'd be taken care of." I chose not to comment on the vagueness of his assurances.

I learned that Molly had grown up in the shadow of her brother Fred, the golden child who had excelled in sports and academics. In contrast to their seeming delight in Fred, her parents, who fought constantly, seemed to regard her as a burden they were forced to endure. Lavishing attention on Fred, they took little interest in Molly's education or in her plans for her future. Although Molly was able to get herself through college and to become a teacher, she regarded herself as a failure in comparison to Fred who had reached great heights in a financially lucrative career.

Molly revealed that she had been mistreated by all the boyfriends she had had before meeting Gene. Never having been regarded as worthy of compassion and understanding, she tolerated varying degrees of abusive behavior from them. Although he never made her feel appreciated, Gene had treated her with a modicum of respect and kindness.

When Gene died shortly after breaking his hip in a fall, Molly was surprised by her lack of sorrow. Why, she wondered, had she shed no tears? When she again mentioned that Gene had not left anything to her in his will, I took the chance of suggesting that she might be too hurt and angry to feel sorrow at losing him. Molly agreed without correcting me. "I am angry," she said, "more than hurt." Then, looking at me intently, she announced, "I have something to tell you that I could never talk about before."

Her confession contained few surprises for me. What was new was her brutally honest self-reflections. She mentioned that Gene's not leaving her money was largely the result of her prideful denials of need. She explained that feeling unworthy of him, she could not make any demands for care and consideration. Never having felt that she measured up to his wife, she accepted whatever he was willing to give her. When he had once mentioned that if they married, she would be left money in his will, she had replied, "We don't have to get married. It's only a formality."

Much as she had longed to marry Gene, she had hoped for a heartfelt proposal in which he declared his great love for her. She needed Gene to want to leave her money. Being a recipient of money because she would be entitled to it as his wife could not satisfy her longing to be experienced as worthy of his gifts. "I felt so ashamed that he didn't love me enough to provide for me," she said.

When I connected her shame at being found inferior to Fred to her shame at the way Gene treated her and her need to assert her worthiness, Molly agreed. At last, her tears began to flow.

As our discussion of a dream that we described in Chapter 3 revealed, her need to be known and appreciated by men began very early in her life. Her father had paid very little attention to her even before her brother was born, and the present he gave her for her graduation her confirmed how little he knew her.

To my surprise it was Molly who mentioned her need to correct me, which, by this time, had disappeared, "I think I found fault with you to level the field between us. You have everything I lack—a career you love, a husband and children." I finally understood that Molly's corrections of me represented her attempt to gain some power in yet another relationship in which she felt as powerless as she had when she was a child. She had clearly envied me.

When I mentioned that I had been deeply troubled by my failure to address her correctly, and that her explanation touched me deeply, Molly again burst into tears. She realized that she had not allowed herself to know that she had exerted power over me. Our discussions helped us both to understand how painful it is to feel powerless in relation to a person we need and how subtle the attempts to wrest power from that person may be. I also realized that I had needed not to know about her envy of me.

Perhaps, Foucault was right about the healing power of confession. It felt as if after our mutual confessions our work together had begun in earnest.

Power and Suffering

Many of us become analysts in order to realize a sense of having the power to heal ourselves or others, power that had been denied us in early life. The more our patients suffer, the more intense the desire to relieve their suffering may become. In this way our patients hold a great deal of power for us. We may gladly give those patients we experience as intensely suffering more of our time and energy than that which we provide for other patients. We may accept lower fees from them or offer concrete assistance to them. Such power is rarely resented because we tend not to feel that we have been coerced.

However, the situation is very different with patients who use their suffering to proclaim their entitlement to our unstinting efforts. They may consciously or unconsciously use their self-perception as victims to try to extract our care. With these patients, we are likely to resent the power we feel that they have over us. We may even engage in power struggles with them and see them as "resisting" the treatment process. We suspect that when we feel "manipulated" by patients it is often in the context of such power struggles.

Jon and Bette

"I have been through the war," Bette complained over and over. She repeatedly mentioned that after her mother had committed suicide when she was ten years old and she had been left in the care of her grief-stricken and preoccupied father. One traumatic experience had followed another. As the victim of what she considered her war-torn childhood, Bette proclaimed her entitlement to flawless responsiveness from me (Jon). After listening to her detailed descriptions about how my last utterance or failure to speak had repeated some childhood trauma, I often felt resentful that she could not appreciate my efforts at empathic attunement. I felt increasingly compelled to serve her ever more perfectly hoping that eventually she would respond favorably.

I now see that Bette and I were locked into a relentless power struggle that was based on what each of us believed to be true. I needed to know that if I responded to her in just the right ways, I would heal Bette's suffering and regain my power as an analyst. Bette needed to know that nothing could heal her suffering; her sense of power was completely dependent on her being the incurable victim.

After some time, I decided to tell Bette that since I was not helping her, she might benefit from working with another therapist. I referred her to a colleague who was considered an expert in working with wartime traumas. After only a few sessions with him, Bette phoned me to say that she was ready to return to analysis with me. Somewhat reluctantly I agreed to work with her again, hoping that she could now appreciate my efforts to help her.

Unfortunately, we soon found ourselves in the same struggle as before. The only difference was that Bette had become more insulting and demeaning in her complaints against me. My efforts to explore what had resulted in her seemingly increased animosity, proved fruitless. Perhaps, she had to fight even harder to maintain the truth of her incurability. At one point, after seeking the advice of several senior analysts, I decided to end the therapeutic relationship. Bette seemed to leave with a sense of triumph—my hardest efforts had not been good enough. My sadness at ending the relationship was outweighed by enormous relief. I wondered if this ending might prove helpful to Bette. Had she finally received confirmation about the dreadful effects of her childhood war zone? I hoped that this might have enabled her to try living without being a victim.

In retrospect, the ongoing battles between Bette and me are also possible to understood in terms of envy. I envied her unabashed identification of herself as being a "war" victim because I still find it difficult to acknowledge the severity of my childhood traumas. She so clearly understood the reasons for her suffering while I had remained uncertain for many years about what had led to mine. Bette seems to have envied me for seeming to have been spared the shameful indignities that she endured. Perhaps, this helps explain her relentless attacks on me.

Clinical Summary

Both Molly and Bette engaged with us in ways that challenged our greatest source of power as analysts: our ability to know how to communicate with patients in ways that we believed promoted healing. Although the outcomes were quite different both relationships illustrated the intense feelings that are generated when this power is compromised. We are convinced that there are as many different ways in which power, envy and relational knowing interact in the analytic situation as there are analytic relationships.

References

Benjamin, J. (1988). *The Bonds of Love: Psychoanalysis, Feminism, and the Problem of Domination*. New York: Pantheon Books.

Benjamin, J. (2004). Beyond Doer and Done To: An Intersubjective View of Thirdness. *Psychoanalytic Quarterly*, 73(1): 5–46.

Brothers, D. & Sletvold, J. (2023). A New Vision of Psychoanalytic Theory, Practice and Supervision: TALKING BODIES. Routledge. New York & London.

Eribon, D. (1991). *Michel Foucault*. Trans. Betsy Wing. Cambridge, MA: Harvard University Press.

Forrester (2017). Foucault, Power-Knowledge and the Individual. *Psychoanalysis and History*, 19: 215–231.

Foucault, M. (1976). *The Will to Knowledge: The History of Sexuality*. London: Penguin Books.

Foucault, M. (1977). *Discipline and Punish: The Birth of the Prison*. (A. Sheridan, Transl.). Random House Vintage Books.

Foucault, M. & Gordon, C. (1980). *Power/Knowledge: Selected Interviews and Other Writings, 1972-1977*. New York: Pantheon Books.

Foucault, M. (1984), *Space, Knowledge, and Power*. In: *The Foucault Reader*, P. Rabinow (Eds.). New York: Pantheon Books, pp. 239–256.

Lichtenberg, J. D. (2024). A Sense of Power: The Motivating Goal of Daily Life. *Psychoanalytic Inquiry*. 44: 791–807.

Silverman, D. K. (2003). Theorizing in the Shadow of Foucault: Facets of Female Sexuality. *Psychoanalytic Dialogues*, 13:243–272.

Vakoch, D. A. (1998). The Therapeutic Space of Psychoanalysis. *Psychoanalysis and Contemporary Thought*, 21: 335–358.

5 Knowing Love and Hate

Love, Plato (1952) tells us, is a divine madness! His evocative description surely conveys something widely shared about the experience that has been given rapturous expression in countless poems and songs. But what is the divine? What is madness? The meanings assigned to these concepts have changed over time and are greatly influenced by culture and world view. Perhaps it is the unique complexity of the feeling known as love that makes it so difficult to pin down with words although attempts to do so have been undertaken since well before the classical Greek period.

Another baffling question is whether we are able to love without being able to hate. Knowing hate is even more challenging than knowing love—especially perhaps for analysts. After all, it is easier for most of us to believe that we love our patients than that we hate them. Convinced that understanding love and hate as both pertain to the psychoanalytic situation is worth the challenges involved, we attempt in this chapter to view them from the perspective of embodied relational knowing. While we examine love before hate, we are not convinced that anyone who truly knows love has not also known hate.

What Can We Know About Loving?

It strikes us as remarkable that even if they are unable to define love precisely, those who feel love seem to have little doubt about what they are experiencing. We humans *know* love. And we also know when it is missing from our lives. It seems likely that one reason for this sort of knowing is that love is a profoundly embodied phenomenon; it exists in exchanges between "talking bodies" (Brothers & Sletvold, 2023). What the bodies of a great many of our patients talk about is their suffering from the lack of love, the loss of love, and/or concerns about their ability to love or be loved.

We are hardly the first to make a connection between knowing and loving. To open several of his books Wilhelm Reich (1933/1949) wrote: "Love, work and knowledge are the well-springs of our life. They should also govern it." Perhaps because Reich was more concerned about sexual experience than love per se, he did not explain how knowledge relates to love.

DOI: 10.4324/9781003487883-6

Erich Fromm was much more explicit about knowing and loving. In an epigraph to his widely read 1956 book, *The Art of Loving*, Fromm cites Paracelsus, a Swiss physician, alchemist, lay theologian, and philosopher (1493–1541), as follows:

> He who knows nothing, loves nothing . . . But he who understands also loves, notices, sees . . . The more knowledge is inherent in a thing, the greater the love.
>
> (Erich Fromm, 1956, p. ix)

For Fromm (1956), love is an attitude of concern that involves the intertwining of care, responsibility, respect and knowledge. He writes:

> To respect a person is not possible without *knowing* them; care and responsibility would be blind if they were not guided by knowledge. *Knowledge* would be empty if it were not motivated by concern. There are many layers of knowledge; the knowledge which is an aspect of love is one which does not stay at the periphery, but *penetrates to the core*. It is possible only when I can transcend the concern for myself and see the other person in their own terms.
>
> (Fromm, 1956, pp. 29–30, parenthesis added)

We believe the knowing that "penetrates to the core" is knowing that involves the whole person; it is a special form of the we-connectedness that we have described (Brothers & Sletvold, 2023) as involving the way bodies talk without words, that is, by means of gaze, touch, tones of voice and so on. Now we would say that when bodies talk, they come to know one another and this knowing, we believe, is a key ingredient of love.

Roger Frie (1997) has called attention to the centrality of love in the work of Ludwig Binswanger (1881–1966), who was a doctor and psychiatrist, but not a trained philosopher. Although greatly influenced by Heidegger's theories, Binswanger criticized them for failing to recognize human sociality. He was more positively inclined toward Martin Buber's understanding of "I-thou" relations. In contrast to Buber, who asserted that I and Thou are separated by the "between," Binswanger understood love relations in terms of a dual "we-hood," a term he used to describe the ontological relation out of which I and Thou first emerge (Frie,1997, p. 93.) Binswanger implies that what humans can know of themselves and one another is based on love.

Believing that the experience of love can only be conveyed nonverbally and extralinguistically, Binswanger turned to poets as "the most competent messengers of love" and asserted that love is most intensely experienced in erotic union" (Frie, pp. 94–95).

Fromm (1975) reminds us that love was not always considered a spontaneous personal experience. Although in most Western societies today, marriages are thought to join loving couples, as recently as the Victorian age, many marriages were based on social considerations; it was commonplace to believe that love would develop after marriage.

Today, the idea that love is a necessity in marriage is probably more strongly held than the idea that love is a necessity in sexual relations. Still, the idea that a loving couple will engage in sexual relations is widely accepted. If embodiment is an important aspect of relational knowing, then the sexually connected loving couple must know one another very well.

We find it interesting that in the Bible, the word "knowing" (*Yada* in Hebrew) is often used to refer to sexual intercourse. For example, in the book of Genesis in the Old Testament, it says, "Adam knew Eve his wife; and she conceived and bore Cain" (Genesis 4:1, NKJV). Here, "knew" implies a sexual relationship between Adam and Eve resulting in the conception of their child.

Many psychoanalysts, following Freud, including Wilhelm Reich, emphasized sexuality over love. Heinz Kohut was an exception. It is interesting to consider the following statement in his posthumously published book:

> It is fruitful to look upon the "I's" experience of the "You" within two separate frames of reference: the experience of the 'You" as selfobject, (the other who is needed to support the cohesion, strength, and harmony of oneself) and the experience of the You as the target of our desire and love.
> (Kohut, 1984, p. 52, parenthesis added)

But then he significantly adds:

> we also realize there are occasions when the I-You experience is most fruitfully approached within a frame of reference that dispenses with the conceptual separation." And he adds: "... object love strengthens the self just as any other intense experience.
> (Kohut, 1984, p. 52)

Here, Kohut reaffirms that it is the connection between "I" and "You" in its various forms that is vitally important and that there are contexts in which people experience themselves and others such that selfobject needs and love may overlap. We imagine that sexuality comes into the picture for him through his mention of desire. We find it interesting that even though Kohut maintains the use of the words "self" and "object" he uses "I" and "You" to explain aspects of a loving connection. (In our 2023 book, we suggested using the words I, you, and we because they allow us to feel their embodied meanings). We also wonder if, with this usage, Kohut was acknowledging the embodied aspects of human connectedness.

Let us return to the relationship between knowing and loving. If loving depends on knowing, then we analysts who are invested in knowing our patients as deeply and intimately as possible, may be uniquely positioned to love them. Jodie Messler Davies (2023) acknowledges the centrality of love in all relationships including the analytic. She writes:

> Do you love me? If there is a foundational human need that immediately follows upon those of food and shelter, is it not the need to know that we are loved?
>
> (Davies, 2023, p. 289)

> Alluding to Fromm's assertion that love is an activity—"a verb not a noun," she suggests that the prototype for our experience of love in adulthood is the childhood experience of receiving unconditional love from one's parents. In development, as receiving love gives way to love based on mutual recognition, a person, she notes, wants to be loved "for my essence, for my uniqueness."
>
> (Davies, 2023, p. 29)

We would say that to be loved for one's uniqueness, one needs to be known as unique. As we have previously suggested, this means being known not as someone who is like any other person but as what we have called "a foreign body" (see Brothers & Sletvold, 2023, Chapter 2). As we mentioned in Chapter 1, we are convinced that humans cannot know one another completely; we confront aspects of foreignness even in our attempts to know ourselves.

Nevertheless, as analysts we develop relationships with our patients that increase the likelihood of our grasping what is unique in them—and, we suggest, they are likely to know what is unique in us as well. Our uniqueness includes the specific ways in which we and they have been "injured, rejected, unloved" (Davies, 2023, p. 291) and, we would add, traumatized. Consequently, loving means tolerating the ways in which these hurtful experiences lead patients to protect against re-experiencing trauma through disengagement, withdrawal—even rage and hatred.

Although analysts expect these reactions from patients, patients do not expect to experience them from analysts. Yet, analysts are just as likely to have suffered from painful traumas and may have to work hard to suppress their own protective reactions that they fear might prove hurtful to their patients. Although patients may deny or dissociate their awareness of their analysts' potentially hurtful reactions to pain and trauma (they may need not to know these things) we believe they do register them in their bodies.

Frie (1997, p. 99) tells us that for Binswanger, the dual mode of love, which he sees as an idealized form of interhuman relatedness, always includes the potential for breakdown. Breakdown, Binswanger explains, occurs when the other is perceived not as an equal subject but as an object to be possessed, be it by domination or adoration. In such cases, according to Binswanger, love may be replaced by hate.

Breakdowns in various degrees of intensity, we believe, are often experienced within analytic relationships although not always with the result that hate is experienced by one or both analytic partners. Although few self-psychologically oriented analysts have focused on analytic hate, preferring to see it as a disintegration product of faulty responsiveness in the caregiving surround, most subscribe to the idea that analytic healing progresses by means of "ruptures and repairs." In other words, they recognize that analysts will inevitably fail to provide the needed attuned responsiveness and that it is only by nondefensively acknowledging these failures that analytic healing can resume.

Our analytic experience confirms the idea that analytic relationships are often deepened and become more growth-promoting following episodes of disruption. As we described in the last chapter, when traumatic memories are triggered for either member of the analytic relationship, power imbalances intensify. In these circumstances the experience of equality and mutuality that Binswanger deemed necessary for the shared experience of dual love may give way to experiences of distrust, suspicion, and yes, even hatred. If not addressed with openness and sensitivity, the analytic relationship may collapse.

It is only when such experiences are given time and space in the analytic dialogue that loving we-connectedness may be restored. Davies (2023) provides examples of loving therapeutic relationships conducted by Steven Mitchell and herself in which the analyst's' reactions to patients who triggered their traumatic memories were acknowledged within healing dialogues.

Yet, despite inevitable disruptions, loving connections often do emerge between analysts and patients. When it does, we can think of no better way to describe it than as Binswanger has; "love is a mutual, unending, giving and receiving" that creates a feeling of "home." (Frie, 1997, p. 96). It is that sense of having found one's home with another person that we believe can make the difference between a healing analysis and one that is not.

Still, most analysts will admit that they do not love all of their patients, even those they know intimately. They simply never feel at home with them. What is it that we know about the other that makes us feel that we make a loving home for them and with them? What is it that they know about us? Binswanger tells us that reciprocity occurs in a love relation when each participant receives "bestowed value" while also bestowing it upon the other. Bestowal of value resembles Kohut's selfobject experience of idealization in which children feel merged with parental figures they view as perfect. Although this sort of idealization experience is thought to dissolve bit by bit over the course of development, and others' imperfections are recognized, Kohut asserts that our need to idealize others endures throughout one's lifetime.

The very notion of idealization suggests that knowing is never absolute or infallible. The mutual bestowal of value between analysts and patient may resemble what transpires between lovers insofar as what is prized in the loved one may not be evident in the eyes of others. Moreover, the idealized bestowal of value may fade or even vanish over time.

Knowing and Sexual Desire

Nothing seems to let us know that we love another person more powerfully than our sexual desire for that person. The embodied intensity of sexual feeling often erases all doubt about our wish to be intimately connected to that person. If we are correct in assuming that knowing that "penetrates to the core" (Fromm, 1956) leads to love between analysts and patients, and if sexual desire leads to a sense of certainty that what we feel is love, it is little wonder that erotic transferences have claimed center stage in much psychoanalytic writing.

Daniel Hill (1994), who celebrates the special place of the erotic transference in psychoanalysis, has traced the evolution of the concept. He notes that the first phase of the development of erotic transferences begins with the difficulties Freud described in the case of Anna O. Freud asserted that the state of being in love which becomes manifest in analytic treatment is not a real one. The professed love, according to Freud, must be exposed as a sham before the analysis can proceed. Yet Freud also recognized the multi-dimensionality of erotic transferences and that the infantile love imbedded in transference love is "real."

Hill views Blum's (1973) idea of a continuum of erotic transferences as representing a second phase in the development of the concept. For Blum, erotic transferences progressively intensify from positive transferences involving affection and friendliness to subtle forms of seduction and finally to "an intense, vivid, irrational erotic preoccupation with the analyst characterized by . . . demands of love and sexual fulfilment from the analyst" (p. 63). Blum saw the emergence of erotic transferences neither as a requirement for analytic success nor a harbinger or its failure.

Hill notes that Roy Schafer (1976) addressed Freud's contradictory views of transference love as real and unreal by suggesting it was both. He credits Ethel Person for appreciating that gender contributes greatly to erotic transferences insofar as it more frequently found in women. Yet Hill says nothing about erotic countertransference.

The relative neglect of literature on analysts' sexual feelings for patients is hardly surprising. While a great many analysts have described erotic transference, far fewer have acknowledged sexual feelings for their patients or erotic countertransference. Among the courageous few are Searles (1959), Kumin (2000), Wrye and Wells (1989) and Davies (1994). Davies (1994) suggests that the difficulties involved in acknowledging sexual longing for patients include the lingering belief in neutrality and abstinence by traditional analysts and an unwillingness by others to view themselves as full participants in the child's romantic oedipal struggles. Celenza (2010) mentions that the power imbalance in the clinical situation, which, she believes, may itself be "sexy," creates challenges for analysts.

There are undoubtedly many reasons for the reluctance on the part of analysts to describe their sexual feelings for patients, or even perhaps, to be aware of them. The history of psychoanalysis may be responsible to some extent. As Aron and Starr (2013) point out, "The talking cure" emerged from Freud's involvement in and eventual rejection of the standard treatment of hysteria, which included stimulating women's genitals by manual and vibratory massage, hydrotherapy or electrotherapy to bring them to orgasm. Moreover, most people feel greatly tempted to act on their sexual feelings and analysts are no exception. The shame and discomfort this arouses for analysts is undoubtedly very strong.

We have wondered if another reason for the difficulty that we analysts face in acknowledging our sexual feelings for patients is that we cannot know these feelings except by tuning into our bodily experience. As we have tried to demonstrate in earlier chapters, when we need not to know on a cognitive level what we know on a bodily level, such knowing is not available to our conscious awareness.

In describing some of the possible reasons that analysts find it difficult to become aware of their own and their patient's bodies in our 2023 book we mention that bodies are subject to immense pain and suffering, and, ultimately, death. We also mention that by focusing on their reactions to their patients' embodiment, analysts are likely to experience unwanted feelings about patients' sex, race, class, culture as well at their physical qualities.

Nevertheless, we feel that much is gained when analysts allow themselves to become aware of their bodily feelings—especially those that are sexual. Since becoming increasingly open to exploring the subtleties of our sexual feelings for patients, we have come to agree with Blum that the range of these experiences is very great. We have found that we sometimes experience tender, rather parental wishes to embrace some patients which involves only very minimal sexual feeling while at other times our feelings are more clearly connected to adult sexuality. We believe that the more acceptable these feelings become the less inclined we are to act on them.

It is often just as revealing to discover that we have no sexual reactions to a patient as to finding that we do have them. Do these patients turn us off in some way? Do they remind us of threatening persons in our own lives? Are they shielding themselves and us from their own sexual desires? The answers to these questions provide important information about the clinical encounter.

In what follows we present clinical examples in which we experienced sexual desire for our patients.

Doris and Dan

It was early in my career when I first met Dan, a 20-year-old student whose chief complaint was extreme anxiety and fear that he would never have sex with a woman. The strength of my positive feelings for him from the earliest minutes of our first session led me to feel confident that our work together would help him overcome his difficulties. I was charmed by his open smile and his direct way of speaking.

Dan explained that while he had always found it easy to make male friends, he had never been able to approach girls without experiencing intense anxiety. As his friends started dating in adolescence, Dan came to believe that something was terribly wrong with him. When well-intentioned friends asked if he might be gay, he felt terribly misunderstood. He knew that he felt attracted to women and had no conscious wish to have sex with men.

We soon came to imagine that Dan's anxiety around women had much to do with his relationship with his aggressive, highly competitive father who seemed to resent Dan's close connection to his mother. Our explorations revealed that his mother had been somewhat seductive with Dan, having allowed him to sleep in his parents' bed whenever he was sick or woke with a nightmare. She had often complained to Dan about his father and seemed to have deliberately provoked his father's jealousy by showering Dan with attention and praise in his father's presence.

I was rather surprised when, after some months of sessions, Dan compared me to his mother. Like her, he thought I was able to "read" his moods and feelings. Although he didn't use this language, he seemed to feel that, like her, I "knew" him. I was even more surprised when he mentioned feeling that I too was seductive. "What makes you think so?" I asked. Dan could not find words to explain what had led him to experience me this way, but he seemed convinced that I was encouraging his sexual feelings for me. "Is this how you think you'll cure me?" he asked.

It was only when Dan announced his conviction that if we had sex, he might overcome his fears about being with women, that the surge of sexual feelings I experienced made it clear that Dan had not been entirely wrong. Although I had not been aware of them, my body must have spoken to him about my sexual attraction to him.

I had little trouble finding a reason for my need not to know my desire for Dan. I realized that he strongly reminded me of myself as young person, fearful of entering the world of sexual relations. Although my story was very different from Dan's, the anxiety I felt had been equally great. Unlike Dan, my reaction was to behave in counter phobic ways. I had plunged into numerous frightening sexual adventures, and I would certainly have benefitted from having an experienced person teach me the sexual ropes. I supposed that if I had become aware of my sexual attraction to Dan I might have re-experienced the anxiety I had felt during this period in my life.

Despite my insight into the reason for my dissociated reaction, I was still shocked by the extent to which I had failed to become aware of my sexual feelings. As we have mentioned in other contexts, we are to some extent foreign bodies to ourselves. We might say that what I knew on a bodily level, my sexual attraction, was not available on a cognitive level. At this point in my professional life, I had not begun to accept even the possibility of having sexual feelings for patients

In response to my telling Dan that I did not believe that our having sex would help him eliminate his anxiety, Dan confessed that he was very relieved. But he still worried that I was turned off by his appearance or manner. Although I assured him that I found him to be a very attractive man, I decided not to tell him about my desire for him for fear that he might experience the disclosure as seductive.

Although Dan made significant strides in the following months in distancing himself emotionally from his parents' marital struggles and was able to establish a platonic relationship with a female student for whom he felt no sexual desire, he could not bring himself to approach women he felt attracted to.

A turning point in our relationship came when a friend told Dan that his girlfriend's roommate was interested in him, and he had given Dan her phone number. "I just can't call her," Dan moaned. "My hands shake when I pick up the phone, and I know I'll stumble over my words. And even if I do manage to ask her out it's bound to be like it was when you refused to have sex with me."

"What was that like?" I asked. "I was really pretty sure that you wanted me, but when you said 'no,' I decided that I must have been mistaken" he responded. He then revealed that he had never known if his mother loved him or if she simply used him as a pawn in her battles with his father. He worried that his ability to perceive a woman's response to him was faulty. "Maybe I just see what I want to see and ignore the truth," he said.

At this point, I decided that it might be helpful to let Dan know that I had desired him sexually. On hearing my words, tears appeared in Dan's eyes. His relief that I had confirmed his experience made me glad I had taken the risk. He then mentioned that he still felt it was good that I had not agreed to have sex with him. "It would have spoiled what we have, wouldn't it?" he said.

It was clear that a significant change had occurred from the moment Dan entered my office for the next session, a broad smile on his face. The woman had called him, and they had met for a drink. "She really seems to like me, and I asked her out for a date this weekend," he said.

Although all did not go smoothly for Dan as he struggled with feelings of distressing ambivalence in his subsequent relationships and sexual difficulties with women, I believe that much healing occurred for both of us. What was particularly helpful for me was that my relationships with Dan allowed me to become more open to my sexual feelings for patients. I would like to think this has been helpful to them as well.

Jon and Jenny

I (Jon) first met Jenny as her training analyst. She had chosen to work with me to fulfill the requirement of my analytic institute that candidates have three analytic sessions a week. In what follows I focus on the loving feelings that developed between us, and the challenges these feelings represented for me.

Jenny, an attractive, clinically talented woman of 30, had not been in a romantic relationship for many years before entering her analysis. When she described having been a very sexually active teenager, I asked her about this seemingly dramatic change in her life. She had no clear explanation for having avoided finding a romantic partner. While she mentioned that her early relationships had not been very satisfying, none seemed to have turned out very badly.

It was not long before I realized that Jenny was becoming increasingly sexually attracted to me. She never spoke of her desire for me, nor did she behave in an openly flirtatious or seductive way. Her long searching gazes and her soft gestures and movements communicated much that she did not say with words. Perhaps, one subtle indication of her desire for me was her repeated insistence that she had no wish to have a boyfriend. However, since she had not put her feelings into words, it was difficult for me to question her about her attraction to me.

To my surprise I soon realized that I was becoming increasingly attracted to her as well. While I never felt tempted to act on my feelings, I wondered what had prompted them. It now strikes me that my longings stemmed from my feeling known by her in a way that met my wish to be experienced as a strong, intelligent, and competent analyst. Perhaps even more satisfying was her obvious enjoyment in looking at me. She clearly found me to be an attractive man.

As time went on our knowledge of one another deepened, especially on a nonverbal level. We both seemed to delight in our contacts especially during silences when we simply looked at one another. In some particularly wonderful way, we had fallen in love.

I became increasingly troubled by Jenny's utter lack of interest in looking for romantic relations outside the therapy room. Our "love affair" seemed to be enough for her. I felt I had to decide whether to tell her that a love relationship—even a nonsexual one—was incompatible with an analytic/therapeutic relationship. Moreover, what we felt for one another might be getting in the way of her finding a life partner. The alternative was to let the relationship develop with whatever feelings might be involve for both of us.

With much hesitation and doubt I chose the latter course. I somehow sensed that treating our feelings for one another as problematic might disrupt what had seemed to be a natural unfolding of our analytic journey.

Eventually Jenny described her relationships with her parents in ways that helped me understand what had attracted her to me. Although she had initially claimed that she had received "good enough" parenting, I learned that her father, an esteemed social scientist, had been very remote. He had seemed peculiarly disinterested in knowing who his daughter was and had never asked Jenny about her studies or her friends. Jenny could not remember having heard any words of praise from him about her appearance or personality. They simply did not talk much.

In contrast, she had had many conversations with her mother. But on reflection, it struck Jenny that their talks had been remarkably superficial. Her mother was concerned with Jenny's choice of clothing and her manners but had never inquired about her feelings.

Jenny had learned about the relational world from reading novels and watching films. She had always had friends but had never found anyone she considered a "soulmate." I was the first person who had really taken an interest in her thoughts, feelings, ambitions and talents. With me, for the first time, she experienced her longings to be known, and I had magically fulfilled these longings. She had also longed to know another person deeply. The closest she had come to such knowing others was in her work with patients.

I came to realize that one of the reasons for our mutual attraction was that I had also felt that neither of my parents had taken pains to know me well or had allowed me to know them. While my parents were quite different from Jenny's in many ways, the similarities had undoubtedly created a special sense of knowing we-connectedness between us. What had stimulated our sexual feelings for one another is part of the mysteries of love that we don't pretend to know.

When Jenny and I were finally able to talk about how our nonverbal connectedness had allowed both of us to feel known, I felt that something important had changed between us. Our sexual desire for one another subsided and was replaced by a sense of being close friends and colleagues. Jenny increasingly discussed her relationships with patients, and I realized that she had incorporated many of the ideas in my books into her clinical work.

Near the time when her training analysis was about to end, Jenny met a man who greatly attracted her. Many of our subsequent sessions were devoted to the development of their romance and love. To my great joy—and relief, they eventually married and now have two children.

When we compare Doris's relationship with Dan and Jon's relationship with Jenny, a major difference between them is that Doris chose to disclose her sexual feelings for her patients while Jon did not. We hope our examples demonstrate that we do not believe that either choice is "correct." We believe when analysts tune into their embodied reactions to their patients, they are more likely to become aware of their sexual feelings. This awareness allows us the freedom to choose to verbalize our feelings or not to do so. We think it is likely that our patients are aware of our sexual feelings even if they are not expressed in words.

Knowing Sex and Gender

There are many people who seem to know without any doubt that they are male or female and that their bodies conform to what their families and culture and religion tell them about these categories. And many people who identify themselves as heterosexual seem to know that they want to be sexual with people of the opposite sex and many who identify as homosexual who seem to know that they want to be sexual with people of the same sex.

However, there are other people who do not know their sex or sexual preference with nearly the same degree of certainty. We like the way Judith Butler (2024, p. 29) writes about them. She says:

> Many endure suffering, ambivalence and disorientation within existing categories, especially the one to which they were assigned at birth. They can be genderqueer or trans, or something else, and they are seeking to live life as the body that makes sense to them and lets life be livable, if not joyous. Sometimes they are living in the interstices opened up between assigned categories and lived modes of embodiment.

We are in full agreement with how she views gender. She writes:

> Whatever else gender means, it surely names for some a felt sense of the body, its surfaces and depths, a lived sense of being a body in this world in this way.

Joan W. Scott (2010) adds that instead of connoting an approach in which the meanings of "men" and "women" are taken as fixed, gender is useful

> if it is taken as an invitation to think critically about how the meanings of sexed bodies are produced in relation to one another, how these meanings are deployed and changed.
>
> (Scott, 2010, p. 10)

These two writers deeply understand both the value of thinking about gender from an embodied perspective and understanding that gender allows us to know ourselves and our embeddedness in our world in ever broadening ways.

We believe that loving others or oneself does not depend on knowing with certainty that one belongs in a specific gender category. Whatever else love is, it transcends knowing what category one belongs in; it is based on one's embodied relational knowing.

Knowing Hate

Throughout the ages, attempts have been made to understand hate by many of the world's leading philosophers, sociologists, psychologists, and psychoanalysts. Yet, even now, there is little consensus on just what gives rise to hatred, what constitutes it, whether the experience of it can be beneficial, and whether it is always present in relationships—even loving ones. For some, hatred leads to conflict and violence. Aristotle, for example, claimed that hate involves the inextinguishable desire to annihilate the hated person. Others have found benefits in hating. Nietzsche asserted that hatred may serve to create needed changes in society.

It is not surprising that Freud, having lived through the horrors of World War I (see Chapter 11), attempted to understand hate from the perspective of his own theory. In a 1932 letter responding to inquiries by Albert Einstein, he wrote:

> *You are amazed that it is so easy to infect men with the war fever, and you surmise that man has in him an active instinct for hatred and destruction, amenable to such stimulations. I entirely agree with you. I believe in the existence of this instinct and have been recently at pains to study its manifestations. In this connection may I set out a fragment of that knowledge of the instincts . . . We assume that human instincts are of two kinds: those that conserve and unify, which we call 'erotic' (in the meaning Plato gives to Eros in his Symposium) . . . and, secondly, the instincts to destroy and kill, which we assimilate as the aggressive or destructive instincts. These are, as you perceive, the well-known opposites, Love and Hate, transformed into theoretical entities . . . Each of these instincts is every whit as indispensable as its opposite, and all the phenomena of life derive from their activity, whether they work in concert or in opposition."*
>
> (Freud, 1932, p. 209)

Ian Suttie vehemently disagreed with Freud's cherished formulations about instincts. In his book, *The Origins of Love and Hate*, which, remarkably, was published in 1935, he courageously took exception to Freud's idea that love and hate are instincts that come into being with the constitution of the ego. For Suttie sociability and love are not derivatives of sexuality. He notes:

> Instead of an armament of instincts, latent or otherwise, the child is born with a simple attachment-to-mother who is the sole source of food and protection... the need for a mother is primarily presented to the child mind as a need for company and as a discomfort in isolation.
>
> (Suttie, 1985, p. 97)

Suttie consequently saw hate as the frustration of love. Hate, he asserted, must be overcome with love by the child. This situation, which removes anxiety by restoring a harmonious relationship between mother and child is repeated in following relationships.

Winnicott's famously addressed the ubiquity of analytic hate in his well-known essay, "Hate in the Countertransference." He writes:

> The analyst's love for his patient is therefore of a very complex kind. However much he loves his patients he cannot avoid hating them, and fearing them, and the better he knows this the less will hate and fear be the motive determining what he does to his patients.
>
> (Winnicott, 1949, p. 70)

Winnicott (1949) adds that psychotic patients cannot be expected to tolerate hate of the analyst unless the analyst can hate them. He emphasizes that analysts must not deny their own hate.

Many contemporary analysts acknowledge the prevalence of hate in analytic relationships as a reaction against more painful feelings. For example, in an

IARPP Colloquium on November 17, 2024, entitled, "On Hatred: Perpetrator Fragments and Totalitarian Objects," Sue Grand wrote:

> As psychoanalysts, we see hatred as secondary to fear and/or shame. I do think that hatred IS a way to escape, and kill off, our vulnerable self states - in particular, aspects of our own helpless dependence. The shaming and repudiation of human dependency is the hallmark of neo-liberalism; it is used to justify starving citizens. This is the ultimate form of disinformation, in which we are trained to mortify ourselves, and our needs, and then, to extrude this mortification into the hated, vulnerable other. And at the same time, to create a channel for dependency in the idealization of a fascist leader.

For Grand, the experience of hating may be extremely desirable. As she explains,

> I would like to suggest that there is something irreducible about hatred, something pleasurable and exciting, that is still not captured by references to shame or fear. I want to suggest that we have difficulty staying with the ecstatic 'purity' of hatred, shifting the focus to hatred's toxicity.
>
> As others have pointed out, it is this ecstatic phenomenon that needs to be understood and experienced, so that we can help our patients with this when it appears in the room. And so that we can accurately reckon with the cultural hatred fomented everywhere.

When hating is considered in terms of relational knowing, we have come to believe that there is often the great disparity between what is known on a bodily level and what is known cognitively--particularly in the analytic relationship. If Winnicott is right that we can no more avoid hating our patients than loving them, we must wonder if that disparity is one of the reasons that the experience of analytic hate is so often omitted from accounts of analytic relationships.

Since relational knowing seems to be largely conveyed between bodies, hate is not a completely well-kept secret between analysts and patients; their bodies speak for them. Subtle changes in the way the bodies of analyst and patient speak to one another—changes conveyed by the tensing of muscles, out-of-sync movements and gestures, and lack of eye contact, are just some of the ways that hate may be conveyed nonverbally.

We doubt that hatred ever arises only because of what is going on between people in the present. The here and now is infused with experiences that have roots in traumas in the hating partners' past lives as well those that have been transmitted through generations. Some experiences of trauma-generated hate represent attempts to reduce life's uncertainty through the insidious creation of an us-them binary that pits country against country, race against race, religion against religion and human against human. When this form of hatred infiltrates analytic relationships, the treatment often unravels.

Doris and Fran

The competitiveness that runs through life in capitalist societies today is particularly evident in the world of publishing. The consolidation of big publishing companies, the high volume of submissions by authors and recent preferences for podcasts and other audio formats over print have made it increasingly difficult for writers of fiction to succeed.

While the insidious effect of this societal situation lies at the heart of my (Doris's) pain-filled relationship with Fran, a middle-aged woman who had written some well-received novels, it was not the only reason that hatred developed between us. She had also experienced crushing feelings of disappointment in me that followed an initial period of intense idealization (Kohut, 1971, 1977, 1984).

When Fran, first uttered words of contempt for me, I was both surprised and shaken. My need not to know that I had disappointed Fran's longing for an omnipotent, omniscient, trustworthy parental figure, was very strong. Nothing in our relationship up to this point, had prepared me for what seemed to be a sudden and unexpected about face in her feelings for me. I now suspect that my longing to continue basking in the praise that she so effusively bestowed on me made it difficult for me to "read" the bodily signs of her incipient hatred before she verbalized it.

Fran had been referred to me by a former patient, an analyst, who had assured her that I would help her overcome a crippling bout of writer's block. We discovered that one source of her difficulties was her very competitive mother who had been forced to end a successful singing career to stay home and raise Fran and her younger brother. Both parents had fallen far short of Fran's criteria for idealization. Her friend's extravagant assurances about my clinical effectiveness seem to have stirred Fran's longing for someone to fill the void in her life.

And Fran did appear to regard me as someone uniquely qualified to help her. Only six months after we began meeting three times a week, Fran began to write again. Our relationship deepened as we explored aspects of her marriage that seemed to replicate her parents' struggles. I felt dismayed by her confessions about her numerous extramarital affairs and the ways she hid expenditures from her husband. Yet, my negative feelings for Fran always seemed to dissolve quickly without my having voiced my concerns. Since Fran had never appeared to feel particularly ashamed or guilty about her betrayals of her husband, I felt unsure about how to convey my misgivings.

Upon the completion of a rather unconventionally told novel, Fran became increasingly disheartened by her inability to find a publisher. She had tried in vain to enlist the help of several well-known agents. It was immediately after she learned that a book of mine had been published that she flew into a rage, "Anyone can write the trivial stuff you put in your book," she hissed.

When I attempted to explore her reaction as a possible reenactment of her rivalry with her mother, she fell into a sullen silence. "Perhaps, it's painful to know that I was able to get my book published when you're running into roadblocks," I ventured. "That's absurd," she snapped. "I write novels and you write gibberish. It's not that you got your dumb shrink book published that's upsetting me, but the fact that you're so damned self-satisfied about it. It's your gloating about your own triumph that's hard to stand." As she hurled these words at me, her tightened features made her barely recognizable.

The sessions that followed brought even more critical attacks about comments that I had made in the past that she now deemed insensitive or misguided. In response to my efforts to apologize for having been hurtful, Fran's attacks became increasingly vehement and personal. It was not long before she announced that she was ending the analysis. She warned me not to contact her. "If I never hear from you again it will be too soon," were her parting words.

It was easy for me to see how Fran's hatred in some way covered her shame over her failure to find a publisher, that she may have envied the apparent ease with which my book was published, and for the power this gave me, but it was hard for me to understand what made her perceive me as gloating over the publications of my own book.

It was only after Fran ended the analysis that I remembered my failure to address what I now realize was my great discomfort about the way she had reported having acted in her marriage. I believe that it was my fear of disrupting her idealization of me that allowed me to overlook her deceptions. Although I never expressed my negative feelings in words, my body must have communicated my contempt for her behavior—my hatred. It is possible that what Fran saw as "gloating" over my accomplishments was my own pride in my own moral integrity compared to hers.

With this realization, I invited Fran to return to examine what had happened between us. She coldly refused, saying that she had found another analyst she could trust. I believe that our relationship might have turned out differently had I allowed myself first to know and fully feel my disapproval when she described her marital infidelity and then had found the courage to speak to her about it. While it is possible that Fran might still have reacted with anger and hostility, I believe it is more likely that she would have valued me as the trustworthy guide she had longed to find. I would have shown myself as someone whose honesty and courage made me someone truly worthy of her admiration. While it is still painful for me to remember how hurt and angry I felt in response to Fran's hostile attacks, I also recall the warm feelings we exchanged in the early stages of our relationship. I terribly regret having lacked the courage to deepen the mutual knowing we needed to heal the wounds of hatred.

Jon and Tom

At times the sources of hateful feelings within analytic relationships reach into the realms of the historical and cultural. Although these sources may be far from either the analyst's or the patient's conscious awareness, they still play a prominent role. This may have been part of the story in the example that follows.

I (Jon) believe that I felt the uneasy stirrings of what led to hate the moment I first laid eyes on Tom. But even as I wrote about my negative reactions to him in a chapter on fascist experience in our 2023 book, I had not allowed myself to feel the intensity of my feelings for Tom until much more time had passed.

On the surface there seemed to be nothing for me to hate about Tom. He is a handsome, intelligent and charming man who is well-respected in his law career. Besides, there was much about him that stirred compassion in me. He suffered from many severe somatic complaints as well as intense anxiety. He had been diagnosed as suffering from PTSD that was based on childhood traumas stemming from his family's frequent moves. His father, who had changed jobs frequently during Tom's childhood, seems to have been indifferent to Tom's needs for stability and safety. He never intervened when Tom complained about being bullied as "the new kid" in class. Tom often said, "my father is a weak man."

As I mentioned in the 2023 chapter, Tom had an oddly elegant manner and way of dressing that called to mind photos I had seen of "Hitlerjugend" (Hitler youth). His arrogant manner, even if understood as defensive, reminded me of the posture of actors portraying World War II Nazis in films I had seen. I realize now that I tried very hard to ignore this troubling association and contented myself with the realization that Tom benefitted greatly from our relationship—at least during the first year of our work together. His somatic complaints subsided, and he seemed less anxious.

Much changed for me when Tom expressed his admiration for Trump and vented anger and contempt at what he referred to as "the extremely stupid liberal and leftwing cultural elite." Being myself liberal and left leaning, I suspected that he knew that I could easily be included among those he despised.

It was not long before our relationship deteriorated and Tom, citing "changed priorities," abruptly left analysis. Here is how I understood my decision not to address the discrepancy in our political views in 2023:

> I was afraid that if I openly voiced my opposition to them, our ***we***-connection would break down. I feared that the analysis would turn into a political discussion and attention would be drawn away from Tom's pressing concerns. At the same time, I wondered if his need for certainty, his maintenance of an "us-them" dichotomy and his antagonism toward political enemies might partially be a consequence of his trauma history.

> Given these considerations, I decided to postpone raising the matter of our political disagreements.
>
> (Brothers & Sletvold, 2023, p. 73)

My understanding today is quite different. I now believe that my need not to know my feelings of hate stopped me from raising our political differences. I believe that it was not so much my hatred of Tom that I feared revealing to him and myself, it was my hatred of all that he seemed to represent for me. I was born only months after the end of World War II and the Nazis, who had occupied Norway during the war, were finally ousted. I have little doubt that my anger and resentment at this horrible time in the history of my beloved country profoundly colored my experience of Tom.

Although I cannot be at all certain, I imagine that Tom's provocative political statements involved, at least to some extent, his wish to test my strength. It is possible that he "read" the bodily signs of my contempt for him before I registered them cognitively. Perhaps he wanted to find out if I was a "weak man" like his father. I now feel that by failing to confront our political difference disappointed Tom's longing to find the strong man he longed for.

Clinical Summary

As we view our past analytic relationships through the lens of embodied relational knowing, it is probably not surprising that those marked by hate stand out very sharply. In the clinical examples we presented, we needed not to know on a cognitive level what we knew to some extent on a bodily level. The tragic consequence of this disjunction in knowing led us to ignore our limitations and vulnerabilities and the powerful effects of the societal factors involved. In both relationships we chose silence over the more challenging option of giving voice to our negative feelings. We realize that the seeming safety of silence often proves to be the more dangerous choice. Still, we appreciate Thato Letsati's (2025) understanding that silence . . . "can shield us from experiences of vulnerability or offer solace and reverence when words feel too fragile."

Despite the pain they have brought us, we are grateful for the valuable knowledge about ourselves that we have gained. We feel better equipped to break the silence that conceals the challenge of both needing to know and not to know the hatred we may feel for our patients. Finding the courage to do so, we believe, will open our hearts to the love and compassion we also feel for them.

References

Aron, L. & Starr, K. (2013). *A Psychotherapy for the People: Toward a Progressive Psychoanalysis*. New York & London: Routledge.

Blum, H. P. (1973). The Concept of Erotized Transference. *Journal of the American Psychoanalytic Association*, 21: 61–76.

Brothers, D. & Sletvold, J. (2023). *A New Vision of Psychoanalytic Theory, Practice and Supervision: TALKING BODIES.* London and New York: Routledge Taylor & Frances Group.

Butler, J. (2024). *Who's Afraid of Gender?* New York: Farrar, Straus & Giroux.

Celenza, A. (2010). The Guilty Pleasure of Erotic Countertransference: Searching for Radial True. *Studies in Gender and Sexuality*, 11: 175–183.

Davies, J. M. (1994). Love in the Afternoon: A Relational Consideration of Desire and Dread in the Countertransference. *Psychoanalytic Dialogues*, 4(2): 153–170.

Davies, J. M. (2023). Reawakening Desire: Shame, Mourning, Analytic Love, and Psychoanalytic Imagination. *Psychoanalytic Dialogues*, 33(3): 69–199. https://doi.org/10.1080/10481885.2023.2204773

Freud, S. (1932). *Why War: A Letter from Freud to Albert Einstein.* Standard Edition, Volume XXII.

Frie, R. (1997). *Subjectivity and Intersubjectivity in Modern Philosophy and Psychoanalysis: A Study of Sartre, Binswanger, Lacan and Habermas.* Boulder Colorado & London: Rowan & Littlefield.

Fromm, E. (1956). *The Art of Loving.* New York: Harper & Brothers.

Fromm, E. (1975). Humanism and Psychoanalysis. *Contemporary Psychoanalysis*, 11: 396–405.

Genesis 4:1, NKJV.

Grand, S. (2024). IARPP Colloquium. *On Hatred: Perpetrator Fragments and Totalitarian Objects* (November 17, 2024).

Hill, D. (1994). The Special Place of the Erotic Transference in Psychoanalysis. *Psychoanalytic Inquiry*, 14: 483–498.

Kohut, H. (1971). *The Analysis of the Self.* New York: International Universities Press, Inc.

Kohut, H. (1977). *The Restoration of the Self.* New York: International Universities Press, Inc.

Kohut, H. (1984). *How Does Analysis Cure?* Chicago, IL; Chicago University Press.

Kumin, I. (2000). On Lust and Loathing: Erotic Transference/Countertransference between a Female Analyst and Female Patients. *Journal of Gay & Lesbian Mental Health*, 4(2): 5–2.

Letsatsi, T. (2025). *Intersubjective Taboos: Finding the Other Within.* Paper presented at a plenary session of the 46th Annual IAPSP Conference, Pasadena, Ca. October 19, 2025.

Plato, 1952. MLA. Plato. Plato's Phaedrus. Cambridge: University Press, 1952. 1956.

Schafer, R. (1976). *A New Language for Psychoanalysis.* New Haven, Ct, & London: Yale University Press.

Searles, H. F. (1959). Oedipal Love in the Counter Transference. *International Journal of Psychoanalysis*, 40: 180–190.

Scott, J. W. (2010). *Gender: Still a Useful Category of Analysis?*

Suttie, I. D. (1985). *The Origins of Love and Hate.* London: Free Association Books.

Winnicott, D.W. (1949). Hate in the Counter-Transference. *Int. J. Psycho-Anal.*, 30: 69–74.

Wrye, H. & Wells, J. (1989). The Maternal Erotic Transference. *International Journal of Psychoanalysis*, 70(6): 673–684.

6 Disorders of Knowing

When viewed from the perspective of embodied relational knowing some common complaints of patients such as those who receive diagnoses of obsessive-compulsive disorder (OCD) and narcissistic disorders take on fresh meaning. Unfortunately, we cannot claim to have discovered new cures for these psychological disorders. Yet, seeing them as disturbances of the need to know, the need to be known, and the needs not to know or be known has led us to develop a novel—and we believe, helpful—clinical approach that entails employing variations of the embodied supervision we presented in our last book (Brothers & Sletvold, 2025).

Obsessions, Compulsions and the Need to Know

A woman is often late to appointments because she feels compelled to check and recheck her stove a great many times before she can step outside. She needs to know that she has turned off the gas burners, but the sense of certainty about having done so eludes her. She is haunted by the fear that a fire may erupt in her apartment at any moment.

An adolescent boy cannot go to sleep until he has repeatedly searched all his social media accounts. He needs to know that he is not the victim of cyberbullying and worries that he will miss evidence that it is happening.

A young mother feels overwhelmed with anxiety unless she holds her newborn son in her arms or sits beside his crib. She needs to know that he will survive but cannot feel certain that he will if she takes her eyes off him.

A 40-year-old man has finally met a woman he feels strongly attracted to but his enjoyment of his dates with her is marred by his need to know that she will agree to see him again. He feels uncertain about whether she finds him desirable until she accepts his next invitation.

Other people repeatedly bite their nails or pick at their skin, take dietary supplements they know are useless, play games on their phones despite feeling they are wasting their time and perform many other unproductive activities ritualistically. They need to know that they have some means of countering otherwise unbearable anxiety even if these activities provide only

DOI: 10.4324/9781003487883-7

minimal help. Still others suffer from not being sure they will not hurt themselves or others, that they will act on sexual or religious taboos, that they will be contaminated by some pathogen. Some hoard material possessions because they never feel certain of having enough.

All these people might be thought of as suffering from some form of the vast variety of symptoms that constitute OCD. As Aaron Esman (2001) has pointed out, although OCD has greatly interested psychoanalysts since Freud's account of the Rat Man, little has been written by contemporary analysts that has added to our understanding of it or has proved curative.

We find that a common thread runs through the accounts of many OCD sufferers: they are unable to feel certain about some aspect of their lives that holds special meaning for them, and they have resorted to employing activities meant to reduce uncertainty. We see a connection between these activities and our understanding of trauma as involving confrontations with profound uncertainty about one's going on being. We have suggested that a reduction of complexity often serves to increase a sense of certainty in the aftermath of trauma—a possible reason that binary thinking is so often found among traumatized individuals (see Brothers & Sletvold, 2025 for other uncertainty reducing strategies). Our attempts to understand OCD disorders have led us to suggest that obsessions and compulsions may also, in certain instances, represent attempts to gain a sense of certainty in the aftermath of traumatic experiences.

Let us take another look at the examples we provided. What we learned about the childhood of the woman who felt compelled to check and recheck the gas burners was that she had been "an army brat" forced to move many times as a child. She never knew for sure when she returned home from school if she would be forced to move again. Her childhood was riddled with traumatic uncertainty. The boy who needed to know if he was the target of cyberbullying, had struggled with an older sister who alternately had been his protector and his rival who would, seemingly without provocation, tease him mercilessly. He could never be certain about "which sister" he would meet next. The young mother who clung to her infant son had experienced several devastating miscarriages and had herself been neglected as a child. She could not bear feeling uncertain about whether she might lose another child or if this child might experience the horror of maternal neglect. The man who could not trust in a woman's wish to be with him had been repeatedly abandoned by his alcoholic mother. He desperately needed to make sure that a woman would not leave him again.

In none of these accounts do we fully understand the link between the traumatic experiences and the development of the OCD symptoms. What triggered the obsessions or compulsions? Why had these people not chosen other uncertainty reducing strategies? We do not rule out the likelihood that constitutional factors played a large role. There may well have been genetic and or other biological factors that predisposed them toward obsessiveness and/or compulsiveness. We have found that psychotropic medications such as SRIs that address the biological aspects of OCD are often beneficial. Nevertheless, we believe that therapeutic relationships may also be extremely helpful. Since the focus of people who suffer from OCD is mainly on their thoughts, we encourage patients like these to become aware of their bodily reactions.

We have found it useful to ask patients to picture themselves back in situations that trigger their obsessions and compulsions. We ask them to focus on what is going on in their bodies at these moments. They usually mention the bodily manifestations of intense anxiety such as racing hearts and rapid breath. In touch with their bodies, they often recapture memories of experiences in which the need to find certainty was great. We then ask them to imagine themselves in the situation again, but this time without enacting the obsessive or compulsive reaction. Repeating this sequence seems to provide patients with the realization that they can do without the compulsive activity as well as a deeper understanding of their own experiences. It sometimes even allows them to experience greater compassion for their suffering.

I-Centeredness and the Need to Be Known

In our 2023 book (Brothers & Sletvold, 2025) we tried to show that I-centeredness (or what are usually called narcissistic disorders) is often the result of efforts to reduce the complexity of lived experience. We suggested that the flow of attention to oneself "I," to the other "You," to the connectedness between oneself and others "We," and to the world—what we call the I-You-We-World flow—is highly complex insofar as it is intertwined with the I-You-We-World flow of others in their relational surround. In the aftermath of trauma, only one of the components may be emphasized as a means of reducing complexity and, therefore the sense of uncertainty. When attention is focused on oneself primarily one is likely to be regarded by others as I-centered.

Self psychologists have referred to such individuals as "mirror-hungry," a result of having been deprived of affirming responses during crucial stages of development. We prefer to think of the experience that was missed in terms of the need to be known. Mirroring, either between parents and children or between therapists and patients tends to emphasize the worthwhileness of the person and their admirable qualities. However, many patients need to be known not only for their admirable qualities and behaviors but for those that are usually demeaned by others.

Doris and Judy

Doris's patient, Judy, a 45-year-old white woman, worked as a high-level executive in a male dominated field. She had come to see me at the recommendation of a male therapist she had worked with for many years. Judy said that she had benefitted greatly from her relationship with him but that he had been too soft on her. When I (Doris) asked her what she meant by "soft," she explained that he had always found a good reason for the behavior that had spoiled a relationship or had gotten her into trouble at work.

What had often gotten Judy into trouble at work was her insensitivity to the needs and feelings of the people who worked under her. Her therapist had tended to empathize with the reasons she had given for her harshness with them. She wondered if, as a man, he might have feared being perceived as aggressive if he had been critical of her. Perhaps, she thought, a woman would be able to lay things on the line about her behavior without worrying about being too aggressive.

I became aware of Judy's I-centeredness early in our relationship. For example, she would insist on changing our appointment time an hour before one was scheduled to begin. When I refused, she would angrily threaten to find a more flexible therapist. Although I never attempted to stop her from doing so, she always phoned for another session a day or so later. When she showed up, I would remind her that she had asked me to deal with behaviors that might be problematic without being "soft" on her. She would usually thank me for being direct and honest with her.

When I asked if she might be willing to explore what had been going on between us from an embodied perspective, she agreed, I suggested that she imagine herself calling to change the appointment time just before a session and to let me know what her bodily experience was. Judy was surprised to discover that she felt tingling in her arms and legs, feelings she associated with being excited and "at risk." When I asked her what thoughts or memories might accompany these feeling, she mentioned seeing herself as a young child marking the kitchen wall with a crayon.

Our exploration of this experience revealed that she had often done what she called "outrageous" things in the hope that she would get her parents attention. She felt that she had been an unwanted addition to the family, born 6 years after the last of her four siblings. "When I did what I was supposed to do, when I was a good girl, I was ignored," she said, "so I did outrageous things. Even if I got yelled at or spanked, I was noticed."

When we worked in a similar way with instances of her harshness with her staff at work, her memories of being a risk-taking teenager and a very promiscuous young woman were revived.

Although we had found a new way to understand Judy's problematic ways of relating, she did not feel that we were excusing her actions. I tried not to let her off the hook about the negative effects of her behavior.

We then began to experiment with her experience of "becoming' the person with whom she had been harsh or unfeeling. To our surprise, tears trickled down Judy's cheeks as she imitated a young employee whom she had berated for what she regarded as her "sloppy work habits." She was flooded with memories of feeling devastated by her mother's fault-finding.

I then asked her to picture the interaction between herself and the employee. Judy was stunned by the enjoyment she derived from what she called "bullying" the younger woman. She realized that she could not focus on the pain she was inflicting. What mattered was the pleasure she felt in being the bully.

Although Judy was grateful for my help in her becoming aware of the negative effect her behavior had on people who worked under her and she was able to moderate her harshness with them, we have been less successful in using this approach in her relationships with her women friends and the men she dates. It seems that when she is in the throes of these complex relationships and flooded with experiences of vulnerability to repetitions of traumatic rejection, she resorts to the I-centered strategies that were once needed for her psychological survival.

Nevertheless, when we examined these experiences together and she has felt known and accepted for her I-centeredness by me, her interest in "living differently" intensifies. I imagine that the more I can focus on how the embodied manifestations of her I-centeredness affects our relationship, the more likely it seems that her personal relationships will improve.

You-Centeredness and the Need to Know the Other

We doubt that we are alone in having begun our training as analysts in our childhoods. Since we felt responsible for the well-being of our parents and siblings, who conveyed their need for us to assume these roles nonverbally, we devoted ourselves to knowing all we could about them. As very young children, we learned to "read" their facial expressions, gestures and tones of voice, etc. for clues to their emotional experience. Even when their words seemed to contradict our findings, we learned to read the "silences between the words." Later as analysts, we drew on this early training in our work with patients.

Jon and Susan

We have found that many of our patients who might be described as pathologically accommodating (Brandchaft, 2007) even those who have worked in the healing professions—were also trained to know others in their early lives. For example, Susan, who has a high position in a prestigious consulting firm, had become expert at knowing her parents as a young child. When her mother fell ill after the breakup of her marriage, Susan realized that her relationship with her father depended on her fulfilling his need that she become her mother's caregiver. Although she could not make time to develop her own friendships and recreational activities, she helped both her parents find new partners. She knew what each was seeking.

It was just her exquisite sensitivity to the needs of her employers that allowed her to achieve success in her career—but at great emotional cost. When she entered analysis with me (Jon), Susan had been suffering from extreme burnout. It became clear that knowing her own needs would have prevented her from being the child whom both of her parents needed. At work, she had also needed not to know about her longing to find loving relationships or even her desire for pleasurable activities. Her only indulgence was food, and she overate without regard to the effects this had on her health.

It was only by focusing on the many ways she had prioritized my needs over her own that Susan began to notice that her standards for meeting others' needs had been impossibly high. For example, she once canceled a doctor's appointment for treatment of a painful skin condition so that she could comply with my request that she change her session time. When I pointed out that I would have tried to find a more convenient time for her had I known about her doctor's appointment, she said: "It never occurred to me to ask you to put yourself out for me." We spent many sessions exploring the reason's this had not seemed possible for her. She realized that her psychological survival had depended not only knowing precisely what others needed, but on attempted to fulfill their needs no matter what the cost to herself or the impossibility of meeting their needs perfectly.

Although Susan is still quite you-centered she has lost a great deal of weight after making time to workout at a gym. Pleased with the change in her appearance, she has searched for romantic partners online. She is now able to point out that although she knows what I need, she manages not to meet my need automatically. In a recent session, noticing that I was not feeling well, she had been prepared to find an excuse for ending the session early. Instead of simply saying that she wanted to leave, she asked how I was feeling. When I told her that I was indeed suffering from a cold but that I wanted to spend the whole session with her, we both felt that we had made considerable progress. Perhaps, Susan knows as well as I, that, like her, I need to feel that I am doing a good job.

Severe Disorders of Knowing

Dementia

Of all the horrible life-ending illnesses we dread—such as cancer or heart disease or any of the countless others that destroy our bodies—we are most terrified of falling victim to dementia, the disease that is thought to destroy one's very sense of self. We doubt that we are alone in feeling this way.

Dementia is the term generally given to a range of conditions that includes the loss of memory, language, ability to problem-solve and fully engage in social relationships. One common cause of dementia is Alzheimer's disease, a degenerative brain disease that is caused by complex changes in the brain resulting from cell damage. But dementia may also result from other conditions such as brain injuries.

The experience of dementia not only profoundly affects its sufferers but also those who care for them. Unlike most other disorders of knowing, dementia often confronts us with a significant before-after dichotomy. The way dementia patients experienced themselves and others—as well as the way others experienced them—before the onset of the disorder is usually greatly different from how it is after it occurs. Since as we have suggested, our relational knowing needs are inextricably connected to our relationships with others, a person to whom we are closely connected who suffers from dementia profoundly affects our need to be known, our need to know others, and our needs not to know or be known.

To illustrate the effects of dementia on the relational knowing needs of those who suffer from dementia and those in their relational surround, we first turn to a book by Mark P. Freeman (2021), *Do I Look at You with Love? Reimagining the Story of Dementia,* as well as a paper he presented at the Psychology and the Other Conference in 2021 entitled, "The Mother of Beauty: Death, Dementia, and the Face of the Divine." In both he describes his experience of his mother's dementia over its 12-year course.

A common response by those witnessing the progression of a relative's dementia was made by Freeman's aunt who said of his mother, "She left us a long time ago." This response, we believe, captures a person's reaction to no longer being known by someone who had once met one's longing to be known. It is often so painful that, for some, it is helpful to think of the person as being "gone" rather than "still here" but no longer able to meet one's need to be known.

At the same time because the person seems so different from whom they were before the onset of dementia, they cannot meet one's need to know them. They are no longer like us and it is difficult to know what their experience is like—especially when the possibility for verbal communication is greatly reduced.

Yet, as Freeman notes, his mother wasn't gone; she had become "scarily other." Although the idea of people suffering from dementia as "other" suggests a harshly dehumanizing view of them he suggests an alternative perspective; as he writes of his mother, perhaps she could be "accepted and affirmed for who and what she's become." He quotes Buber (1965) as follows:

> This person is other, essentially other than myself, and this otherness of his is what I mean, because I mean him; I confirm it; I wish his otherness to exist, because I wish his particular being to exist. . . . That the men with whom I am bound up in the body politic and with whom I have directly or indirectly to do, are essentially other than myself, that this one or that one does not have merely a different mind, or way of thinking or feeling, or a different conviction or attitude, but has also a different perception of the world, a different recognition and order of meaning, a different touch from the regions of existence, a different faith, a different soil: to affirm all this, to affirm it in the way of a creature, in the midst of the hard situations of conflict, without relaxing their real seriousness, is the way by which we may officiate as helpers in this wide realm entrusted to us as well, and from

> which alone we are from time to time permitted to touch in our doubts, in humility and upright investigation, on the other's "truth" or "untruth," "justice" or "injustice."
>
> (pp. 61–62)

Although we could not even hope to express this idea as eloquently as has Buber, it is our belief that like all other humans, people suffering from dementia need to have their unique humanness known

> We have found that a body-based approach to working with these patients has enhanced our ability to welcome their otherness. That is, our knowing needs and theirs are met less with words than with embodied forms of connectedness. We find support in Fuchs' (2021) understanding. He contends that although dementia robs patients of their explicit memories, they still retain their bodily memories which includes their familiarity with environments and habits as well as their sensory and motor memories. He contends that instead of relying solely on rationality and autonomy their sense of self is based on intercorporeality and interaffectivity.

Our first clinical example illustrates this phenomenon.

Jon and Allen

Allen, a 30-year-old veteran, began analysis with me some years after I had completed working with his mother. Although he had found his combat experiences as part of a Norwegian peace-keeping force in Lebanon difficult, Allen had taken pride in having come through the physical and psychological challenges relatively unscathed. He was highly articulate and engaged me in interesting conversations about how his combat experience had made him feel different from his friends who had not served abroad. He also spent much time talking about his relationships with women.

After a year of sessions, he seemed to have made considerable progress in analysis. He expressed greater satisfaction in his work as an accountant and seemed pleased with a new relationship. Most importantly he had begun to make plans to leave his parents' home and to rent a small apartment in another part of the city.

When he failed to show up for a scheduled session, I phoned his home. His mother answered, tearfully explaining that Allen had suffered severe brain damage in a horrible auto accident and was still recovering in a hospital. Some months later, she called to ask if she could take Allen to a session to see me. Although Allen looked much as before, he seemed to have been replaced by another person. Walking unsteadily and looking bewildered, he seemed to be extremely childish and insensitive to the usual protocol of the treatment situation. Although he spoke rapidly and continuously, it was extremely difficult to follow him. He seemed not to have remembered who I was or what our relationship had been about.

It was not long however before Allen began to repeat the bodily behaviors that had marked sessions before the accident. He chose the chair he had used although others were available. He tapped his fingers on the armrest as he had always done. And soon he clearly seemed to recognize me and to remember that we had had a relationship earlier. After some months, Allen was able to speak coherently despite problems with both his long- and short-term memory. As his ability to recall events that happened the day or so before returned, he would report in great detail what had happened with little regard for its relevance to our work.

It was only when he stopped talking that our connection seemed to resume something of the way it had been before the accident. I could tell by the way he looked into my eyes that he had feelings that he could not find words to express. I learned that my efforts to find words to capture what I imagine was going on for him were not helpful. It was only when we were able to connect silently that our feelings for one another seemed to flow.

There are times now, when I feel bored and impatient in sessions with Allen as he relates, in painstaking detail, some new interest of his that holds little meaning for me. Yet, I am gratified by the realization that since he is no longer able to work or even to leave his parents' home unaccompanied, my listening is important to him. And then there are the precious moments of silence that we share when our un-worded feelings flow freely in a way that renews our deep connection.

Doris and Stella

In earlier chapters we have mentioned that there are times when the needs to know and be known intertwine with the needs not to know and not to be known. The slippage between knowing on a bodily level and not knowing cognitively is especially pronounced in those suffering from dementia. But it is not just the dementia patient for whom knowing on a body level differs from what is known on a cognitive level, it may also be true of the therapist. Doris's experience with Stella is illustrative.

Stella sought analysis with me when she was 80 years old. She had finally "had enough" of the neglect and abuse her male partner, Ed, had been subjecting her to for many years. He had called her "stupid," "ugly" and (worst of all, according to Stella) "old" during their frequent fights. Why had she put up with him for so long? What had she ever seen in him? What was the power he had over her?

Growing up in a loud, fun-loving, earthy family, Stella had always felt loved but somehow different from all the others. What did she see in poetry and art, she was asked. Why didn't she play sports like her siblings. She had married a "nice" man but someone who seemed to fit better with her siblings than with herself. When he died and she was introduced to Ed, he seemed like the answer to her prayers—at least for a while.

Our explorations revealed that Ed was the only person she had known who had truly appreciated her aesthetic sensibility and her dry sense of humor. With him she felt deeply known for the first time in her life. When she displeased him—a frequent occurrence—she could not discount his cruel remarks as untrue. After all, he saw the best in her, perhaps, he also saw the worst. It was only when his hurtful words were accompanied by slaps and shoves, that she decided to seek help in leaving him

Stella mentioned that Ed's rageful attacks occurred whenever she had turned her attention away from him. "I want to be me without worrying about how that affects another person," she said. Within months of sessions, she asked Ed to leave. Although he pleaded and threatened her, she remained firm in her stance.

After several weeks of tearful reminiscences of the tender moments she had shared with Ed, Stella seemed almost reborn. "I feel stronger and happier with myself than I ever imagined possible," she said. "I thought that Ed understood me, she said, but his understanding had strings attached. He understood and accepted the parts of me that benefitted him. He hated the parts of me that were for me." Then she said. "Doris, I don't think you pick and choose the parts of me that suit you. And you always let me know there's more to me to discover." I could not have been given a more meaningful tribute!

The following year brought many positive changes in Stella's life. She joined a book club and wrote poetry again. She also reconnected with a daughter who had withdrawn from Stella's life when Ed had moved in with her.

I'm not sure how I could have missed the unmistakable signs of Stella's incipient dementia for the many long months in which they had become increasingly apparent—but I did. Perhaps it was because I had felt so delighted in how she seemed to know and find words for just how I helped her that I failed to notice her deteriorating memory and cognitive abilities. It was only after she entered my office, near the end of the usual time for a session, in a very agitated state, explaining that she had gotten lost on her way to my office, that I realized how much I had needed not to know about her deterioration. Although she had mentioned misplacing her belongings and forgetting the names of friends, I had attributed these deficits to the ordinary sequela of aging.

As the symptoms of her dementia worsened, Sheila repeated stories she had told me many times. She missed more appointments than she kept. She withdrew from her book club, complaining that she could no longer follow the discussions. And most painfully for her, she stopped writing poetry. Alarmed, I asked Stella how she understood these changes in her functioning. "I'm still me," she said, "but I'm afraid that you think I'm losing my mind. "I admitted feeling very concerned about her and suggested that she consult a neurologist. The results of the exam were distressing to both of us; Alzheimer's disease was suspected, and she was given symptom reducing medications including Aricept.

Once the tentative diagnosis had been made and even though her prognosis was grim, she seemed relieved. "At least I know what's happening to me," she said. I, on the other hand, had a much harder time accepting the inevitability of her decline. In contrast to those who regard a person suffering from dementia as "gone," I clung to my belief that Stella was still "here." I even imagined that the diagnosis was incorrect and wondered if her symptoms might reverse. For several months, I tried to conduct sessions with Stella as usual. Because her memories for past events remained intact, I would listen quietly without saying that she had already told me most of these stories before.

Eventually, however, I could no longer avoid fully accepting her deteriorating cognitive abilities. The more I faced the reality of Stella's cognitive decline, the freer I seemed to become to feel my love for her. I believe that Stella responded to the change in me as well. Speaking had become increasingly difficult for Stella. She would begin a sentence and become unable to find her way to the end of it. We enjoyed long periods of silence. I say enjoyed but the quality of the intimate connectedness we experienced without words is indescribable. For long moments we simply gazed at one another. At times she would take the hand I extended toward her. And occasionally she would stroke my arm or my hair.

Eventually, Stella could no longer come to my sessions unattended. She was accompanied by an aide her daughter had hired to care for her. After some months, Stella's daughter asked to speak to me. She mentioned that she could not provide all the home care that Stella now required and that she had arranged for her to be placed in a care facility. I was heartbroken. Although, I told Stella I would stay in touch by phone, it was not long before she could no longer manage the conversations in which I did the talking. We both seemed to feel that these conversations fell far short of the silent hours we shared in my office.

The call that I had been dreading came a short time later. Stella's daughter let me know that she had suddenly died of a stroke. With the diminution of my initial grief, I was left with a powerful sense of gratitude that I had shared the precious moments during the last part of Stella's life with her.

Although I feel some regret that I had not recognized the early signs of her dementia, I cannot be sure that it would have changed very much between us. I have rarely experienced a richer sense of we-connectedness than I did in the silence of my last moments with Stella.

Our relationships with Stella and Allen have convinced us that what we cannot know though verbal exchanges with dementia patients can be reached in silent communication. And perhaps our knowing needs are more richly filled when our bodies and not words do the talking.

Madness—Rational Knowing and Nonrational Knowing

Although Freud (1905) doubted that psychotic patients could benefit from psychoanalysis insofar as what he called their "narcissistic defenses" would prevent them from establishing transference relationships, he acknowledged that "suitable changes" in his method might "succeed in overcoming this contra indication—and so be able to initiate a psychotherapy of the psychoses." We will not attempt to name all the many notable analysts throughout the history of psychoanalysis who attempted to develop such changes in method.

Our efforts to understand what we prefer to call madness in terms of its effects on the relational knowing worlds of patients perceived of as mad and those who are connected to them has led us to turn to a variety of psychologists, psychoanalysts and philosophers. We have turned to the writings of George Atwood (2011), whose phenomenological contextualist approach allowed him to reject a view of view psychosis as a medical disease. Instead, his clinical work reveals how the traumatic loss of human connectedness gives rise to the relational manifestations that are deemed psychotic.

Our understanding has also been informed by the neuroscientific and phenomenological work of Vittorio Galese, Martina Ardizzi and Francesca Ferroni (2024). Contrasting their view with that of contemporary organistic psychiatry which emphasizes abnormalities in neurotransmitter systems as well as other neuroscience perspectives that neglect the experiential dimension of psychotic disorders, they view schizophrenia as "a self-disorder characterized by anomalous self-experience and awareness" (p. 152). They develop a new "embodied cognition" approach that views schizophrenia in terms of a disrupted connection between and individual's bodily self and the social environment. We find similarities between this perspective and our idea disruptions occur between what is known on a bodily level and known and not know on a cognitive level.

As Daniel Posner (2024/25), who also subscribes to a phenomenological perspective, writes: "The current phenomenological model situates the core self-disorder in schizophrenia as a disturbance in "ipseity." Ipseity, for Posner (2024) refers to "the foundational self-affectivity or "self-presence" that gives our experience its cardinal sense of "mine-ness"—the "first-person" (Stanghellini & Lysaker, 2007). In Sass & Parnas' (2003) original ipseity-disturbance model, attenuation of "the minimal self" can be thought of as the ontological origin of a range of inter-related self and intersubjective disturbances unique to the schizophrenic spectrum condition.

Hannah Lyn Venable (2022) has helped us to see that the phenomenological approach to madness, as developed by Merleau-Ponty and more recent thinkers, which posits that madness is intrinsic to human experience, should be integrated with Foucault's archaeological-historical perspective, according to which madness arises out of cultural structures. While for

Merleau-Ponty, madness is a subjective state that must be understood in its own terms, he also observes that madness uses the structures of the world. In this respect his understanding resembles Foucault's. Both philosophers have fought against the view of rationality as distinctly different from nonrationality that has prevailed since the time of Kant and Descartes.

Venable (2022) observes that a consideration of both the phenomenological and the archeological "points to the integration of the rational and the nonrational" (p. 29). We find her assertion that the nonrational can never be entirely severed from the rational to be particularly illuminating with respect to embodied relational knowing insofar madness has been historically understood in terms of irrationality. She writes:

> The reliance on the nonrational . . . is not something found only in abnormal behavior but in all human behavior. Thus, whatever value we attribute to a distinctively human way of interacting with the world, we must attribute to both functional and dysfunctional ways of experiencing the world in the sense that it remains human. The value of humans placed in normal and abnormal categories is equal because of the shared way we encounter the world.
>
> (Venable, 2022, p. 226)

Venable's perspective aligns with Atwood's insofar as his book represents an attempt to "erase the sharp boundary that has been drawn to separate madness from sanity, returning the phenomena of severe psychological disorders to the circle of the humanly intelligible" (2012, p. xii). He asserts that "... individuals we consider insane are simply human, all too human" (p. x1).

We agree that the need to know and be known does not only pertain to what is considered rational, but also to the nonrational. We have not found criteria that can distinguish between what is rational and nonrational when we consider that both kinds of knowing may be intensely longed for. We reject any suggestion that the analyst's need to know and not now pertains only to the rational while the mad patient's knowing needs pertain only to the nonrational. Such a perspective tends to silence the nonrational aspects of human experience. We are more concerned about the extent to which we as analysts can accept the patient's needs as validly human.

We strongly agree with Venable's contention that the integration of the rational and nonrational is only possible because the mind cannot be separated from the body. She quotes Merleau-Ponty as follows:

> Mind is not a specific difference which would be added to vital or psychological being in order to constitute man. Man is not a rational animal. The appearance of reason and mind does not leave intact a sphere of self-enclosed instincts in man.
>
> (Merleau-Ponty, 1963, p. 181)

In the *History of Madness*, Foucault (2006) traces the history of what he calls unreason or (*déraison*) through the Renaissance, the classical age, where he locates the beginnings of the complete alienation of the irrational, to the modern age. As Venable (2022, p. 106) notes, "Due to the irrational being ignored by society and exiles, there is a 'rupture in dialogue' between the rational and irrational; the irrational is then 'reduced to silence' and upon arrival of the modern age, its voice can no longer be heard." She cites Foucault's (2006, p. 56) conclusion that even today, "... unreason remains mute, and forgetting comes from the great silent wounds within man" (p. 56).

As Venable (2022), drawing on Foucault, notes:

> The ignoring of the irrational shifts the way those labeled mad are handled in the modern age. No longer a constructive reminder of the irrational as in the sixteenth century and no longer hidden away in the seventeenth and eighteenth centuries, they are now seen as people who have deviated from the normal standards of society and need to be fixed, through both ethical and medical means, so that they can be brought back into society.

For us, seeing madness in terms of the mad patient's needing to know and not needing to know as including both the rational and nonrational helps us to avoid trying to "fix" them by insisting that they become normal. We believe we are likely to be far more helpful if we acknowledge that their ways of knowing are valid.

Jon and Mandy

I (Jon) first met Mandy, a 25-year-old single woman, shortly after she had been released from a psychiatric hospital where she had been diagnosed as schizophrenic—a diagnosis she almost proudly embraced. "I hear voices and have trouble thinking," she explained. But when Mandy described the neglect and abuse—both sexual and physical—she had experienced throughout her early life, my impression of her psychological difficulties had less to do with madness than with severe trauma.

Mandy had not chosen me to be her therapist but had been referred to me by the hospital's administrators. Yet, she accepted me as her therapist without complaint and she showed up on time for her twice-weekly sessions. Her need to be known by me seemed much greater than her need to know me since she evinced little interest in my life. Rather she seemed to relate to me as a replaceable professional, one in a long line of therapists she had seen over the years.

She spoke in heartbreaking detail about her abuse at the hands of her alcoholic stepfather and other men in her life. She also complained about acquaintances whom she experienced as insulting and rejecting. Although she is quite attractive, she is considerably overweight. One man who had been a sexual partner but had stopped being sexual with her because, he said, he was "turned off by her fat belly," was one of her few friends.

It was not until she reported hearing sounds of people having sex through the walls of her apartment and spoke of "just knowing" that neighbors were talking about her in negative and crudely sexual ways that I remembered her diagnosis. She is also convinced that aliens from outer space inhabit our world.

Initially, I thought that I had only two choices: I could simply listen quietly to what seemed like delusional stories (her nonrational way of knowing) and hope that my presence as she related them would comfort her, or I could let her know that I doubted their veracity. If I listened without comment, however, I imagined that she would "hear" my body talking about my disbelief.

At some point it occurred to me to try to provide an alternative understanding. I suggested to Mandy that there might be another way to make sense of what she had been hearing, and I asked her if she wanted to know what I had in mind. Mandy agreed. To my surprise, she became very interested in my suggestion that the sounds she heard through the walls of her apartment had reminded her of her experiences of sexual abuse. Perhaps, I added, she had elaborated these sounds into a narrative that had elements of her own sexual experiences. Mandy seemed relieved to think that she was not once again at the mercy of hostile others as she had been as a child.

When she reported that others had been rude or insulting to her in situations in which there seemed to be alternative ways of understanding them, I asked her if we might be able to imagine the situation from the perspective and bodily manner of the other person. Again, Mandy was intrigued. I discovered that she was remarkably skillful at imitating the insulting person's facial expressions, bodily gestures and tones of voice. During these exercises, Mandy seemed to quickly grasp that she was not deliberately targeted for abuse. However, her understanding seemed to resist generalization from one situation to the next.

Despite Mandy's enthusiasm for these new ways of experiencing, she has not relinquished what might be thought of as her nonrational narratives. It has become increasingly clear to me that much as she is able to understand what might be thought of as her symptoms of madness in terms of my traumatic interpretations, she still clings to her own experience of herself as the victim of others' malevolence—and she continues to report these experiences to me without any suggestion that they might be understood differently.

Perhaps it is only in my presence that Mandy can relinquish her experience of being subjected to the malevolence of others. But I have little doubt that she finds my acceptance of her—as she is—an important and healing antidote to her suffering. She seems to feel known by me as an intelligent, sensitive woman who has a place in my world.

As we have attempted to understand Mandy's experience in terms of embodied relational knowing we believe that she both needs to know that she is the victim of the malevolence of others and, at times, in the presence of a trusted therapist, that others mean her no harm. In line with Gallese, Ardizzi and Ferroni (2024) and Posner (2025), we imagine that disturbances in her sense of embodied wholeness lead her to switch from one way of sensing herself in relation to her surround to another quite completely.

We imagine that Mandy's reluctance to relinquish her sense of continual victimization represent the failure of witnessing by others at the time of her abuse. She may hope that if her current accounts of abuse are accepted as true, her life narrative has validity and that she is entitled to compassion and acceptance for her suffering. Still, we believe she has benefitted from her remarkably successful efforts to take the perspective of others. The quality of her relationships with people in her social surround seems much improved. Her circle of acquaintances has widened, and she enjoys outings and meals with others. What we and others deem nonrational has important meaning in her life.

Summary

Our understanding of the ways in which a therapeutic perspective based on embodied relational knowing is helpful in treating severe disorders of knowing—such as dementia and madness—is very much in keeping with our approach to the concept of the "Other." In a symposium at the 2025 Psychology and the Other Conference that we participated in entitled, "Otherness in Question: Embracing our Shared Humanness in Encounters with Dementia and Madness, we wrote;

> we must embrace one another as "Other," as unique individuals who cannot be completely known. We must heed Levinas' warning against reducing the alterity of the Other to sameness. In fact, we must re-evaluate the very meaning of "Other" and apply the concept to include ourselves.

While we try to apply this understanding to all our therapeutic relationships we realize that doing so is particularly challenging in our encounters with patients suffering from severe disorders of knowing.

References

Atwood, G. E. (2011). *The Abyss of Madness*. New York and London: Routledge, Taylor & Francis Group (Psychoanalytic Inquiry Book Series).

Brandchaft, B. (2007). Systems of Pathological Accommodation and Change in Analysis. *Psychoanalytic Psychology*, 24: 667–687.

Brothers, D. & Sletvold, J. (2025). Embodied Relational Knowing with Dementia Patients. Paper presented at Psychology and the Other Conference symposium, "Otherness in Question: Embracing our Shared Humanness in Encounters with Dementia and Madness". September 17, 2025.

Buber, M. (1965). *Between Man and Man*. Ronald Gregor Smith (Ed.). Collier Books, 1965.

Esman, A. H. (2001). Obsessive-Compulsive Disorder: Current Views. *Psychoanalytic Inquiry*, 21: 145–156.

Foucault, M. (2006). *History of Madness*. Trans. Jonathan Murphy and Jean Khalfa. London: Routledge.

Freeman, M. P. (2021a). The Mother of Beauty: Death, Dementia, and the Face of the Divine. Presentation at the Psychology and the Other Conference. Boston, MA.

Freeman, M. P. (2021b). *Do I Look at You with Love? Reimagining the Story of Dementia*. Rotterdam & Boston: Brill/Sense.

Freud, S. (1905). On Psychotherapy (1905 [1904]). *The Standard Edition of the Complete Psychological Works of Sigmund Freud*, 7: 255–268.

Fuchs, T. (2021). *In Defense of the Human Being: Foundational Questions of an Embodied Anthropology*. Oxford: Oxford University Press.

Gallese, V., Ardizzi, M., & Ferroni, F. (2024). Schizophrenia and the Bodily Self. *Schizophrenia Research,* 269: 152–162.

Merleau-Ponty, M. (1963). *The Structure of Behavior*. Trans. Alden L. Fisher. Pittsburgh, PA: Duquesne University Press.

Merleau-Ponty, M. (2012). *Phenomenology of Perception*. Trans. Donald A. Landes. London: Routledge.

Sass, L. & Parnas, J (2003). Schizophrenia, Consciousness, and the Self. *Schizophrenia Bulletin*, 29(3): 427–444.

Stanghellini, G. & Lysaker, P. H. (2007). The Psychotherapy of Schizophrenia Through the Lens of Phenomenology: Intersubjectivity and the Search for the Recovery of First- and Second-Person Awareness. *American Journal of Psychotherapy*, 61(2): 163–179.

Venable, H. L. (2022). *Madness in Experience and History: Merleau-Ponty's and Foucault's Archaeology*. New York and London: Routledge.

7 Knowing Couples

We could not begin to provide a complete list of all the reasons couples give for seeking therapy to help their troubled marriages or relationships. Illnesses—both physical and mental, losses, traumas, infidelities and developmental imbalances are just a few we have heard. Yet, no matter what has gone wrong, we believe that viewing relationships in terms of embodied relational knowing may help clarify the nature of the difficulties couples encounter and point toward directions for healing.

When couples first meet, their needs to know one another and to be known are usually very strong. In addition to wanting to know about one another's background, relational history and present livelihood, they often formulate questions that are rarely voiced. Will they be loved and accepted once the new person comes to know them? Will the new person provide the developmental experiences missed in their early lives? Will the new relationship provide safety and stability or painful repetitions of ones that ended badly?

Couples often find some of the answers to these questions in the ways their bodies communicate. When our patients talk of "chemistry" between them and their partners we know they are referring to much more than simply sexual attraction. Clearly, what they know on a bodily level may not be known on a cognitive level. Even when the words exchanged are exactly what each wants to hear, their bodies may "know" that all is not well. An averted gaze, an impatient gesture, a tense smile, a clenched muscle may say what words cannot. But a gentle touch or smile may also send important messages that cannot be spoken.

Since bodies communicate between couples in very intimate ways, we have found that employing an embodied approach to therapeutic work with them has been helpful. As our examples will hopefully illustrate, our therapy with couples also makes use of the approach we use with disorders of knowing (see Chapter 6) that derives from our model of embodied supervision (Chapter 9). For example, we may ask couples to get in touch with bodily feelings at times when we notice that their emotional experience seems to have been neglected in their spoken dialogues. Doing so often provides new information about what is being communicated that may otherwise be

DOI: 10.4324/9781003487883-8

overlooked. At other times we may ask them to "become" their partner by imitating the partner's expressions, gestures, bodily movements, and ways of speaking. This often allows them to understand the feelings that had given rise to hurtful words spoken or actions taken by their partners. Occasionally, we may ask each member of the couple to form an image of some embodied interaction. These images often reveal surprising aspects of the relationship that have remained out of awareness.

Just as embodied supervision often reveals what is going on between supervisee and patient in ways that we could not have known, so embodying the therapeutic process with couples often provides understanding that we could not have reached on our own.

The interplay between the need to know and the need not to know is often apparent in the relationships of new couples. Unwilling to diminish the blissful delight of being in love, some may be only too willing to keep their eyes closed to aspects of the new person that might tarnish the relationship.

In Chapter 2 we discussed how secrets may reflect the need not to be known, noting that most people keep some thoughts, feelings, ideas, etc. to themselves. We noted that when the needs not to know or be known are unconscious, they may represent dissociated experiences, Secrets, on the other hand, are usually conscious. Relationships between couples are frequently disrupted when secrets become known—especially secrets involving sexual infidelity. The following clinical example is illustrative.

Jon and Sara and Erik

Sara had seen Jon for individual therapy for many years during which she had not mentioned difficulties in her marriage. She had sought his help for traumas related to the suicides of family members as well as conflicts with co-workers in a stressful work environment. Five years after ending individual therapy, she asked Jon if she could return for couples therapy with her husband. Jon agreed to see them together.

Jon soon learned that Erik, Sara's husband had become hostile and withdrawn after Sara had told him about her sexual relationships with men she had met before she married Erik. Why on earth, she wondered, was Erik upset about her disclosures. She had been completely faithful during their marriage.

As Jon explored the context for Sara's descriptions of her earlier relationships, he discovered that Erik had been critical of Sara's appearance since she had gained weight after the birth of their second child. Jon had not known that Sara had always struggled with her weight; she had kept it a secret. She tearfully explained that after Erik had refused to have sex with her, she had told him about torrid sexual experiences in her pre-marital life in the hope of reviving his desire for her.

Wishing to increase Erik's emotional understanding of the context of Sara's disclosures about her pre-marital sexual experiences, Jon then asked Erik to "become" Sara by imitating her expressions, gestures and way of talking. After imitating Sara for several minutes, Erik began to understand how shameful and distressing her weight gain had been for her. He told her that he was sorry for turning away from her just when she already felt unlovable.

When Jon then asked Sara to "become" Erik, she understood that he had interpreted her weight gain as a rejection of him and as indifference to his needs. She remembered that Erik had told her that when his younger sister was born, his mother had abruptly turned away from him. Sara apologized for having so completely shifted her attention from him to her new baby.

Jon encouraged them to form an image of their interactions around Sara's disclosure of her sexual experiences. It became clear to them that Sara's having had sexual relations with men before meeting Erik was not what had upset him. Nor was her graphic account of them the main reason for his distress. They realized that the disruption in their relationship had much to do with what they had not wanted to let one another know: their vulnerable and shameful feelings of being unlovable and unworthy.

Doris and Maya and Barry

While disruptions of relational knowing mark the painful disconnectedness faced by most couples who seek therapy, they are probably most intense among couples who come from different ethnic, cultural and/or class backgrounds. Because couples tend to wish to be known and to know the other in terms of the cultural language in which they were raised, they often feel that their needs have been neglected by partners who have not learned the "grammar" of their native cultural tongues.

That was at least part of the reason that Maya and Barry, fearful that their marriage was breaking apart, sought Doris's help. During a blissful honeymoon period both had felt as if they had never been known more deeply and completely. Their delight in deepening their connectedness ended abruptly when Maya's parents, who were born in a southern Asian country, both fell ill. Maya could see no alternative but to move to her parents' home to care for them. In her culture, the expectation that children return home under such circumstances was experienced as a moral obligation. Although Barry understood why Maya's parents would not hire expert nursing care, he resented having to move to the distant state in which they lived. Reluctantly, however, he agreed to leave a place he had come to feel would always be their home.

Almost immediately, Maya seemed to change from the kind, agreeable woman he thought he had married into someone who was angry, demanding and continually fault-finding. Feeling that his needs were neglected in favor of Maya's parents', Barry withdrew from her emotionally and recoiled from her physically, no longer providing the affection and consolation that Maya had come to expect from him.

Exploring the dramatic reversal in their relationship with Doris, it became clear that Maya had always been known by her parents and siblings as the "difficult" child. Despite having a graduate school education, and finding work in a demanding profession, she was often demeaned and criticized for any perceived misstep or failure. Barry was the first person to have acknowledged Maya as the kind, helpful person she had wanted to be. Maya saw his withdrawal as evidence that he shared her parents' negative perception of her. How could he not see that her behavior was consistent with the role she had been assigned in her family, she wondered. Didn't he know that she couldn't behave differently when she was living under their roof?

Barry's early life had also been filled with challenges. His father had moved his wife and 5 children repeatedly because of business opportunities that rarely materialized. Always feeling that they were the outsiders, the family had closely bonded with one another. Negative feelings were disavowed not only because they augured disintegration of much needed closeness but also because their religious upbringing had foregrounded the expression of love and gratitude.

With Maya's insistence that they move, Barry had re-experienced the traumatizing effects of his childhood dislocations. But he had been unable to express his anger at this repetition without violating the family taboo; withdrawal was his only refuge.

When asked to "become" Maya, Barry trembled and shook his head. "I can't," he said. In reply to Doris's questions about what he was experiencing, he said he felt that he was choking. Asked to try to stay with the choking feeling just a bit longer, he began to weep. After a few minutes, he said that perhaps he had always choked back his anger, an acknowledgment that represented a major step forward in their therapy.

Maya had little trouble imitating Barry. Smiling sweetly and speaking in a soft, gentle voice, she said, "I'm a good son and husband who never has an unkind word to say." Then she said, "Oh, I think I'm caricaturing Barry." Barry stopped her, "No, you've got me." I do exaggerate my goodness-which means being a person without anger."

There was no need to ask them to form an image of their interaction. It had become clear that, under the stressful conditions of life with Maya's parents they had assumed the opposing roles they had needed to play in their early lives.

It was not easy for either of them to relinquish their accustomed ways of relating but they reported being increasingly able to recognize bodily signs indicating that dysfunctional patterns were repeating. They have become better able to avoid the painful impasses that had threatened to end their relationship, and they share more moments that recreate the intimate knowing that marked their early years.

Sudden Differences

Couples often seek therapy after one of the partners suddenly changes. An Illness, accident or precipitous life choice may alter the various aspects of relational knowing for the one who changes as well as the one who has remained relatively the same. Those who change may feel unknowable, sometimes even to themselves, while their partners may feel betrayed by the disruption to their sense of knowing. In extreme cases, these changes are experienced as traumatizing insofar as the couple is suddenly confronted by enormous uncertainty about a relationship that had once been their anchor.

One change that profoundly disrupts a couple's relationship occurs when one of the partners suddenly becomes cognitively impaired. In Chapter 6 on disorders of knowing we mentioned the profound disruptions of relational knowing that occur among dementia patients and their loved ones. The sense of loss for both members of a couple when one develops dementia can be overwhelming. Even when the cognitive decline is relatively mild for one partner, it can result in painful disruptions in relational knowing for both.

This was true for Alan and Debra. Although the onset of Alan's Parkinson's symptoms such as tremor and fatigue had been rapid and severe, the couple's relationship had seemed to deepen as they learned to cope with Alan's physical limitations. But when Alan developed difficulties with his short-term memory and executive functioning, Debra reported feeling as though she was living with a stranger." "I don't even want to touch him," she admitted.

Debra had depended on Alan to organize their daily lives. She was happy to have him manage their finances, decide what plays and movies to watch, where to go on vacations and what restaurants to visit. She even left decisions about the timing and manner of their lovemaking to him.

With the realization that she would have to assume an active role in managing their affairs, she not only lost the sense of knowing Alan, but she also felt that she did not know herself either. Having been an overburdened child in a large family, she had relished feeling like a pampered child in their marriage. She had not wanted to know that she could take responsibility for anyone or anything.

From the beginning of their life together, Alan had been only too happy to be the one in charge. Growing up in the shadow of a brilliant older brother, he had thoroughly enjoyed being "the big man" for Debra. Her withdrawal from him had overwhelmed him with feelings of inadequacy much like those he had experienced in childhood.

When they sought couples therapy with Doris, both could not imagine life without one another but since their life had changed so dramatically, they could no longer imagine a shared future. Realizing that Alan was unable to express his feelings in words very easily, Doris turned to Debra. Asking Debra to say what she experienced in her body when she looked at Alan, Debra mentioned feeling that all her muscles were tense. Noticing her clenched fist, Doris asked her to focus on it. "I'm so angry," she exclaimed. "I hate that Alan can't take care of me anymore. I hate myself, too, for still needing to be treated like a child." Then as her body relaxed, she said, "I love Alan and want to help him. I don't know what to do."

Noticing Alan's expression of dismay at hearing Debra's words, she asked Debra to "become" Alan by imitating him. Wrapping her arms around herself as Alan had done, she said, "I feel so small and alone. I need to be close to Debra again."

Alan then said, "I don't want Debra to do everything herself. But I can't do everything I used to do for her." In response to Doris's questions, it became clear that Alan could still make many of the decisions about their recreational and cultural life as he had before. Debra expressed relief, realizing that she had exaggerated the extent to which Alan could no longer take part in their life. She said, "Maybe it's about time for me to become an adult. I don't need to be Alan's little child anymore." As she spoke, Debra took Alan's hand. "I've missed us," she whispered. Alan smiled for the first time in weeks.

By the time their couples therapy came to an end, Alan's condition had stabilized, his cognitive functioning had not worsened, and new medication had lessened his tremor. However, both Debra and Alan acknowledged the likelihood that Alan's illness would progress at some point. They expressed hope that they would be able to face whatever the future might bring with grace and acceptance. They spoke of learning to cherish the moments of tender sharing that occurred more and more often between them and that they seldom succumbed to despair about the inevitable hardships they would endure in the years ahead.

We hope these examples of embodied relational knowing as it applies to therapy with couples will inspire others to further explore and develop this approach. There are undoubtedly ways to modify our style of working that will prove useful for difficulties between couples that we have not encountered.

8 Knowing Communities

Auguste Rodin sculpted his famous "Thinker" as a nude male figure, his chin resting on his hand, seated alone on a bare rock. He is presumably lost in deep contemplation. The sculpture masterfully expresses a widely held belief that thinking is a solitary process, the results of which are the thinker's sole creation and possession.

We could not disagree more. Although we often experience thinking as something that goes on in our minds alone, what is revealed when we think about ourselves, others and the world is greatly influenced by the accumulated knowledge of others—past and present. In this chapter we try to show that our needs to be known, to know others and not to be known or to know are also greatly affected by our embeddedness in familial, cultural, ethnic, religious, professional and friendship communities. Some knowing communities serve to promote our development and healing while others are extremely detrimental to our wellbeing.

Usually, one of our needs for embodied relational knowing assumes greater prominence than the others. At any given point in time, our need to experience the sense that we are known may be greater than our need to know another person. Or our need not to know becomes more urgent than being known or knowing. The intensity of one of these needs is undoubtedly affected by the relational context in which we find ourselves, which includes the needs that are experienced by one's relational partners and communicated both with and without words.

But there are times when none of the aspects of embodied relational knowing gains ascendence. While not being aware of the urgency of one or another of one's embodied relational knowing needs may indicate contentment and equanimity, it may sometimes reflect a loss of connection with one's sense of self—or one's sense of being out of sync with others, even with one's analyst. These are often the times when our patients report feeling stuck. We hear them say: I can't find a way to go forward in my life, or I can't find the courage to leave my marriage, or I can't stop overeating or drinking, or I can't finish the book or paper I'm writing.

DOI: 10.4324/9781003487883-9

Sometimes analysts are the ones who feel stuck—sometimes because of a conflict about needing to know how to help their patients and needing not to know something about them or themselves that is getting in the way of their knowing. Often, the way out of the sticky place for both patients and analysts involves finding the right community of knowers. For example, analysts are often helped to become unstuck in their work by members of their supervision groups. Knowing communities can also be immeasurably helpful for patients.

Doris and Rick

Upon selling a lucrative business that he had poured his heart and soul into creating, Rick, a 45-year-old white man, complained that his life had lost meaning. His need to be known as a high-functioning man who had been successful in all his previous professional and personal enterprises became apparent early in our first session. He was, he announced, self-made and self-sufficient. His only reason for seeing me, he claimed, was that he needed professional help to find a new project worthy of his talents and skills.

As we continued to meet, he reluctantly confided that his solution to what we identified as ungrieved loss, not only for his beloved business but for missed emotional experiences in growing up with mis-attuned and somewhat neglectful parents, was to drink excessively.

He also admitted that while he had always found his wife wanting as an emotional and intellectual partner, he enjoyed her beauty and her sophisticated taste in home furnishings, art and clothing. Most of their shared moments involved drinking either by themselves or with their friends. Rick had wrapped himself in the persona of "the party guy" who could drink everyone else "under the table." Yet, he confided that his heavy drinking had led to explosive bursts of anger that were endangering his friendships and his already shaky marriage.

Nothing seemed to change in Rick's life for many months and although I was gratified by his increasing trust in me, my confidence in my ability to help him develop new interests or even to reduce his heavy consumption of alcohol began to fade. We were both feeling stuck. It was only after he called me for a session from a hospital bed where he was being treated for severe pancreatitis that the gridlock began to give way. Frightened by the seriousness of his illness, he confessed. "I can't keep up this charade. I'm not able to stop drinking on my own." When he asked if I thought Alcoholic Anonymous (AA) might help, I encouraged him to give it a try.

Up to this point, I had attributed my not suggesting that he join AA to his repeated assertions of self-reliance. I told myself that he would scoff at the idea of joining any sort of helping group. But I have come to realize that my need to be known as a self-sufficient healer matched Rick's need be known as totally self-sufficient businessman. I had wanted to help him resolve his problems without assistance from others. Perhaps we had both been seduced by the societal attitudes that inspired Rodin's solitary thinker.

Although Rick's participation in AA meetings did not help him to discover a new professional endeavor, he experienced great relief and comfort in being among people who were struggling with similar problems. After experiencing how generously members of the meetings he attended met his need to be known, a need that had been unmet most of his life, he realized that he had gotten used to feeling lonely, unknowable. Rick was particularly moved when, after speaking about his shame at succumbing to the urge to drink again, many in his group spoke of their own shameful failures. That others could allow him to know them in their painful vulnerability was also a startling realization for him. Befriending some like-minded AA members, he reveled in their intellectual companionship and soon reduced his contact with people who had supported his "party guy" persona.

We were now able to address long-standing problems in his marriage. When I suggested that he and his wife consult a couples therapist, he readily agreed. The idea that help could be found in community was now something he endorsed. No longer the self-sufficient knower, he asked me for help in finding a bereavement group for his mother when his father died after a long illness.

We believe that one of the reasons for the success of healing communities like AA is that they provide a sense that one's needs to be known and to know others are shared and amplified. One is no longer alone with a seemingly intractable and insoluble problem. Our patients have identified many helpful knowing communities such as those formed by writing groups, fine art groups, dance and recreations groups, meditation and yoga groups. For analysts, supervision groups are particularly helpful knowing communities (see Chapter 9).

Knowing Therapy Groups: The Power of Witnessing

Having led therapy groups for many years, we are convinced that the degree to which relational knowing needs are met within a group greatly influences the healing that occurs for its members. That is to say that therapy groups serve as knowing communities.

Simply discovering that others are trustworthy knowing partners is meaningful for many group therapy patients. But perhaps an even more important way in which the healing process occurs in groups is by means of witnessing. Both the experience of having one's painful experiences witnessed by others and by serving as a witness for the pain of others promotes healing for many patients—especially those who have failed to receive confirmation for their sense of reality.

In each meeting of Jon's therapy groups using a method developed by choreographers Diane and Albert Pesso (Pesso & Crandell (Eds.) 1991), resembling aspects of Moreno's psychodrama, patients were chosen to play roles in one patient's life while the others served as witnesses. Consider Henry's group experience: 44 years old, married, and the father of two boys, Henry had been raised by well-meaning parents who nevertheless had neglected his emotional needs in favor of his older sister's. She had been born with a devastating medical condition and needed constant attention. Even after Henry had been bullied by a troubled classmate, his pleas for attention and comfort had been ignored.

Jon selected several group members to act as Henry's parents and sister. He asked them to ignore Henry while he tried to elicit their attention by recounting his ordeal of being beaten outside of his school. Others in the group then reported on what they witnessed, staying as close as possible to his emotional experience. One of the group members asked Henry if his parents might have attended to him had he chosen a time to report on his distress when they were less concerned about his sister. Henry then was able to play a scene in which his parents responded sympathetically to his plight. Henry realized that he often replayed the earlier scenario in his own family when his wife was busy with their children. He realized that he had often chosen times to ask for help from others when they were not receptive. His experience had reinforced his idea that his needs could not be met, a way to have his early suffering known.

As this example illustrates, the role-playing method that Jon used consisted of two parts. In the first part, group members enact a scene that recreates the negative aspects of a member's family dynamics and in the second part, they enact one in which a more positive result is achieved. Because the other group members serve as witnesses to both the painful aspects of the member's experience and to their finding a possible solution, they gain by imagining how the situation might apply to their own lives.

Doris's therapy groups, which began early in her career, have not been organized around a specific approach but rather have integrated aspects of various psychodynamic perspectives that have changed over time. While she had first adopted a radically non-directive approach in which she believed that what emerged in the group should not be determined by her influence, she has come to view herself as playing an inescapably powerful role. She believes that her needs and feelings are expressed in an embodied way that often "speak" to the group members without words. The members of her groups have either ended individual therapy with her or continue to see her individually. During the group meetings, she sometimes chooses to interact directly with a patient while at other times, she asks the other group members to respond to what a patient provides.

Gina, a 30-year-old woman, joined one of Doris's groups while continuing in individual therapy which she had begun several years earlier. She had been raised in a prominent family in which one's worthiness was measured by material wealth and professional status. She doubted that she could be known for any of her qualities that did not show up in her bank account or in the title after her name. As she increasingly risked revealing herself and her feelings in the group, many of the members appreciatively responded to her empathic sensitivity and humor. She delighted in being known as someone whose emotion-laden responses to the distress and joy of others in the group allowed them to feel deeply known.

Although Gina had discussed the emotional brutality inflicted by family members in her individual sessions, she had not initially risked revealing it to the group. After witnessing other patients' accounts of being emotional wounded by family members, she began to disclose her own suffering. As group members responded with compassion, Gina provided increasingly harrowing details of being both physically and emotionally tormented. After many months, in which she voiced anger toward her parents and siblings for their unfeeling brutality, she explained that she had finally stopped excusing her family's hurtfulness in the belief that she "deserved it."

Gina noted that she not come to this realization in individual therapy. It was only after witnessing the unprovoked hurtfulness that others in the group had suffered and through their compassionate witnessing of her suffering that she came to understand that she had not "asked for" her abuse. She also came to realize that by claiming responsibility for her own suffering she had been able to maintain her connections within her family. She had believed that since they were so accomplished and admired, people outside the family could not measure up to them. She had consequently made few friends and rarely dated. The group had taught her, she said, not only that she could be accepted by people who did not judge her by what she had earned but that she valued others for the very qualities she wanted known about herself.

Charles, a 60-year-old man, received word that a CT scan had showed a recurrence of his cancer. At the time of his first cancer diagnosis, Charles had been a new member of the group. He seemed to react to his condition with remarkable acceptance. He made many statements to the effect that he was lucky to have lived as long as he had and to have had many "blessings." However, when his cancer returned after the initial treatment had produced a near-total remission, Charles learned that the group members really wanted to know what the experience was like for him. His psychological well-being as one of six children had been maintained through his "not making himself a bother" for his overwhelmed parents. It was stunning for him to realize that his not being a bother would have deprived group members a chance to know what this terrifying experience was like and an opportunity for them to show their support and love.

We have not begun to describe the many different kinds of groups that serve as helpful knowing communities. However, as we attempt to demonstrate in what follows, we also feel it is important to examine knowing communities that bring pain and suffering to their members.

Destructive Knowing Communities

That the intense need to belong to knowing communities sometimes results in tragedy is horrifically exemplified by the People's Temple cult that formed around Jim Jones in Jonestown, Guyana. Survivors told of being beaten, humiliated and brainwashed into signing their possessions over to Jones. On November 18th, 1978, following the shooting of Leo Joseph Ryan, Jr., a US congressman who had come to investigate the compound, Jones ordered 900 of his followers to swallow a fruit drink laced with cyanide, sedatives and tranquilizers. All of them died. Jones himself died of a gunshot wound (Gunn, 2017).

What members of the Jonestown cult had in common with members of other destructive communities, many of which might be called fascistic, include obeisance to an all-knowing leader, beliefs that are not supported by scholarly research (conspiracy theories), and a sense of being under threat from those outside the community.

One of the hallmarks of these cults, and the reason that we designate them as knowing communities, is that they form around powerful leaders who claim to have knowledge that their followers lack. These leaders deliver simplistic messages that often stir deep feelings in their followers, feelings that are usually deemed unacceptable by those outside the group. Accepting the wisdom of the leader's emotional massages, members experience a sense of being united by their shared beliefs and devotion. Safety, they believe, lies within the confines of the knowing community; dangers lie outside it.

Heinz Kohut (1971) taught us we never outgrow the need for contact with those who serve as idealizing selfobjects, a need that originates in early childhood. Such figures are experienced not only as omnipotent but also omniscient. By experiencing ourselves as merged with these figures, often our parents, we gain a sense of partaking in their guiding, protective strength. Although the idea that these figures are unfailingly omniscient is usually outgrown by the end of adolescence, the longing for such figures can be revived in the context of trauma. This is undoubtedly one of the reasons that a charismatic leader who asserts his omniscience is particularly appealing when the world seems most chaotic and turbulent. In this era when the planet itself appears close to destruction and violence has erupted in many places in our world, it is hardly surprising that we are vulnerable to those Kohut (1978a 1978b, p. 823) called "charismatic and messianic personalities." These leaders, whom he notes, "display apparently unshakable self-confidence and voice their opinions with absolute certainty," qualities he suggested that exquisitely meet the needs of their followers, those who "long for merger with all-powerful and all-knowing ideal figures" (1969–1970/1978, p. 108).

In earlier writings (Brothers, 1995, 2008; Brothers & Sletvold, 2023) we have stressed the importance of the fascistic leader's certainty when the world is trembling with uncertainty. While we still believe that leaders' expressions of certainty are important to their followers, we now appreciate how their assertions of being all-knowing exert an equally powerful appeal. When we struggle to understand political and cultural upheavals in our world that threaten our survival, we may long to re-experience the safety and protection offered by an omniscient parental figure. Donald Trump appears to understand this longing well. He often tells his audiences that his is very smart and that he has all the answers to their problems. His messages are simple and often involve appeals to the us-them binary.

How is it possible that cult members do not know how harmful their leaders are? We suspect that even among the most devoted of a cult's followers, some glimmers of knowing that the leader may be hurtful and destructive may become conscious at times. However, it seems to be characteristic of cults that while not knowing and knowing may coexist to some extent their need not to know greatly outweighs their need to know.

Our patients have let us know that families sometimes have the characteristics of destructive knowing communities. Growing up with a tyrannical parent (usually a father) who asserts his omniscience can leave children with life-long deficits in their sense of their own ability to know. We think of Carol, a 50-year-old woman Doris treated, whose father was a well-known surgeon. He made no effort to mute his contempt for the intellectual shortcomings of everyone in his family. Although Carol's mother and brothers were often targets of his criticism, his attacks on Carol, who suffered from ADHD, were brutal and relentless. She remembered feeling that since he was brilliant and well-respected in the community, she must be as stupid and incapable of achieving professional success as he repeatedly asserted.

Luckily Carol was a talented athlete who gained admission to college on a sports scholarship. Despite having done well enough academically to graduate from college and having found employment, she remained convinced that she was intellectually inadequate. "Everyone knows how to live happy lives, except me," she repeated mournfully. She felt certain that the reason for her relational difficulties, particularly in romantic relationships, was her lack of intellectual ability.

Increasingly however Carol has accepted evidence that her failed romances are attributable to her finding critical men like her father in the hope that she could reverse her painful past; this time, she hoped, the critical man would come to know her as intellectually competent and thereby provide some counter measure to her father's demeaning judgment.

Carol is beginning to understand how difficult it has been for her to relinquish her belief in the negative judgments of the men she has found. As someone presumably unable to know, she maintained her connection to her father which was based on his need to demonstrate his superiority. In addition, by celebrating her husband as "a genius" whose wisdom could not be doubted, Carol's mother had modeled the need to rely on a strong male knower.

In her therapeutic relationship with Carol, Doris has been careful not to undermine Carol's belief in her father. Doing so would have simply created a situation in which Carol had to choose between Doris' wisdom and her father's. Nevertheless, as Doris acknowledges Carol's gains in understanding her psychological world, Carol has taken a number of bold steps toward living her life as an intelligent woman. She has even started writing a screenplay.

The Psychoanalytic Community

Analysts and other mental health professionals have not been immune to powerful temptations either to become leaders of knowing communities themselves or to become followers of such leaders. While much good has come from these knowing communities, including important theoretical and clinical advances, it is hard to find psychoanalytic institutes and organizations in which conflicts both within the group and outside the group have not caused suffering for participants. Much has been written about the harm inflicted by such infamous therapeutic cults as the Sullivanians (Stille, 2023) and Feeling Therapy (Brothers, 2003, 2008). Phyllis Grosskurth's book, *The Secret Ring* (1991) reveals that such conflicts existed among Freud's early followers as well.

We believe that there are signs that psychoanalysis has begun to overcome its insularity and infighting. In recent years the internet has provided analysts with opportunities for knowledge of all kinds to be shared by means of podcasts and online conferences that reach across the borders of individual countries, Moreover the topics that now appear in leading psychoanalytic journals reflect a growing willingness to discuss political and economic upheavals and conflicts. Let us hope that psychoanalysis will increasingly model a knowledge community that provides a sense of we-connectedness to all who share its spirit of inquiry and scholarship.

References

Brothers, D. (2003). Clutching at Certainty: Thoughts on the Coercive Grip of Cult-like Groups, *Group*, 27(2/3): 79–88.

Brothers, D. & Sletvold, J. (2023). *A New Vision of Psychoanalytic Theory, Practice and supervision: TALKING BODIES*. London & New York: Routledge.

Grosskurth, P. (1991). *The Secret Ring: Freud's Inner Circle and the Politics of Psychoanalysis*. Reading, MA: Addison-Wesley.

Gunn, J. (2017). *The Road to Jonestown: Jim Jones and Peoples Temple*. New York: Simon & Schuster.

Kohut, H. (1971). *The Analysis of the Self: A Systematic Approach to the Psychoanalytic Treatement of Narcissistic Personality Disorders,* New York: International Universities Press.

Kohut, H. (1978a). Psychoanalysis in a Troubled World. In P. H. Ornstein (Ed.), *The Search for the Self: Selected Writings of Heinz Kohut: 1950-1978*, vol. 2, (1978). New York: International Universities Press, pp. 511–547.

Kohut, H. (1978b). Creativeness, Charisma, Group Psychology: Reflections on the Self-analysis of Freud. In P. H. Ornstein (Ed.), *The Search for the Self: Selected Writings of*

Heinz Kohut: 1950-1978, vol. 2, (1978). New York: International Universities Press, pp. 793–844.
Pesso, A. & Crandell, J. (Eds.) (1991). *Moving Psychotherapy*. Brookline Books.
Stille, A. (2023). *The Sullivanians: Sex, Psychotherapy and the Wild Life of an American Commune*. New York: Farrar, Straus & Giroux.

9 Knowing Supervision

If, as we have tried to demonstrate in the preceding chapters, approaching therapeutic relationships from the perspective of embodied relational knowing reveals much that might otherwise have been overlooked, it may be even more illuminating with respect to the supervisory situation. In this chapter we describe how we have added aspects of embodied relational knowing to the model of supervision that we have been developing.

As we have continued to experiment with this updating of our supervision model, our belief that clinical knowledge and authority reside mainly in the bodies of supervisees and their patients rather than in the theory or clinical experience of the supervisor has grown even stronger. In fact, we have found that a consideration of the knowing needs of supervisees and their patients allows for a deeper appreciation of the idea that we meet one another as "foreign bodies" (Brothers & Sletvold, 2023) who cannot be completely known. Much as asking questions about their patients' (and their own) needs to be known, to know others, and not to be known or to know others provides more information about the therapeutic relationship, it also confronts the supervisee with the limitations of therapeutic knowing. Yet, this awareness does not seem to increase a sense of hopelessness about the healing potential of their therapeutic relationships. Rather we have found that many supervisees who have confronted the humbling limitations of their knowing seem to have gained compassion for themselves and their patients. In addition, suggestions by other group members of a range of possible ways to "know" their patients confirms the idea that there is no correct way to engage therapeutically. Space is left for surprise, playfulness and experimentation within the therapeutic relationship.

Let us begin by reviewing the supervision model we described in our 2023 book:

> We start by asking supervisees to provide a brief account of the patient and the progress of the therapeutic relationship as is often done in traditional

DOI: 10.4324/9781003487883-10

supervision. We then ask them to state what it is that they would like to explore in their work with the patient they have presented.

Next, we ask them to assume what we refer to as the ***"I"*** position. In this position the supervisees imagine being in a recent session with the patient. They are asked to "see" the patient again and to describe what they feel in their bodies when they do so as well as any thoughts, images, fantasies, etc. that arise.

Then we ask them to assume the ***"you"*** position. Here they are asked to "become" their patient. They do so by imitating the patient as closely as possible. They are prompted to imitate the patient's facial expressions, gestures, ways of sitting and moving and even speaking. (Nebbiosi and Federici (2008, 2022) describe imitating their patients following sessions in a way that resembles this position.) Next the supervisor addresses the supervisees as if they were the patient. The remarks made to the patient vary greatly depending on what the supervisors feel may be pertinent to the situation presented.

We want to emphasize that we do not believe that when the supervisee "becomes" the patient, what emerges is the truth about what the patient is experiencing. Rather it is what the supervisee has unconsciously felt that the patient is experiencing.

In the ***"we"*** position that follows, the supervisees are asked to reflect on the interaction between themselves and their patients while remembering their experiences in the ***I*** and ***you*** positions. We have often found that new ideas about what has been going on in the therapeutic situation emerge at this point. Supervisees may then be asked if they would like to experiment with their new understanding by imagining themselves to be with the patient again. Sometimes this involves changing their posture or distance from the patients, or the way they speak. But often this simply involves feeling something new about the situation.

When supervision is conducted in a group setting, ***world*** enters the supervisory setting more explicitly. As we see it, this occurs as the other group participants bring their own unique flow of ***I-you-we-world*** to the therapeutic situation presented and thereby increase the complexity, richness and even the beauty, mystery, and uncanniness for the supervisee.

After completing the ***I-you-we*** positions, the supervisee is asked to imitate the patient once again for a short time. All the other participants in the supervision group are instructed to *"become"* the therapists for the patient presented and to first attend to what they experience in their bodies, then to notice what feelings, thoughts, images, and fantasies arise for them. They are instructed not to attempt to "supervise" the supervisee but to direct their comments to the supervisor. They may be asked to explain how they would work with the patient. The supervisee is often asked to comment on what each group participant contributes.

(Brothers & Sletvold, 2023, pp. 78–86)

Introducing Embodied Relational Knowing

When embodied relational knowing is added to the supervisory relationship, the supervisor asks the supervisee questions related to the supervisee's own knowing needs and those of the patient. Because these needs are often partly unconscious, we ask supervisees about what they *want* to know or not know, which is usually conscious, and not what they *need* to know.

In the "I" position, after supervisees describe their embodied reactions to a patient, the supervisor asks the following questions: "What do you want to know about your patient? What do you want your patient to know about you? What don't you want to know about your patient? What don't you want your patient to know about you?"

The same questions are then repeated in the "**you**" position except that they are asked of the patient whom the supervisee has "become" though imitation. It is understood that the answers given reflect the supervisees' sense of the patient since they have no way of knowing what the patient would actually have replied.

Let us provide some examples from the supervision/study group we conduct monthly with a group of trained clinicians from a variety of countries and theoretical orientations. Since meetings of this group take place on Zoom, we have been able to record the meetings and then to transcribe them. In what follows we use portions of these transcriptions that we have minimally edited in the interests of clarity. To protect the patients' confidentiality, we use only an initial for the supervisee's name and we refer to their patients by the name the supervisees gave them.

We start with a detailed description of a supervisory experience in which a very experienced clinician felt that he had lost the capacity to work with one of his patients.

G and Elaine

In his brief description of his troubled relationship with his patient, G explained that Elaine, an intelligent 18-year-old woman had sought therapy with him after cutting herself and attempting suicide. Confiding that she had been too ashamed to let anyone else know what she had done, she told G that it was a relief to confide in him. Elaine's self-attacks had followed a profound betrayal of her trust when she discovered that the man with whom she had fallen deeply in love was a pimp. G also mentioned that after her parents divorced, her father had stopped paying for her schooling. Elaine's troubled relationship with her father was another source of her distress.

Asked what had led him to request supervision, G said: *"I feel totally at a loss—empty. And Elaine feels empty to me. My capacity to work with her has disappeared."*

When G mentioned that in the last session Elaine hadn't made eye contact with him, the supervisor (Jon) suggested that it might be helpful for G to try to recapture the experience of being with Elaine in the last session.

In the "I" position, after Jon asked G to report on what he felt in his body when he imagined being back in the last session with Elaine, G replied:

> *It's difficult to breathe. My belly is very tense and something scary is going on in my head. It's like I'm losing control, and I have no words. The only word that's coming to me is "desperation".*

G seemed to have experienced his bodily pain as caused by his belief that he had lost the ability to help Elaine.

In answer to Jon's question, "What do you want to know about Elaine now?", G answered:

> I would like to be able to go very, very deeply to the place inside Elaine where she's crazy. There's a place inside her—it's a dark place with no light inside. I would like to be able to see where she's crazy. It's very scary but I would like to go there.

G had not realized that he had experienced aspects of Elaine's experience as psychotic. He also understood that he was not afraid of connecting with her when she was psychotic.

In response to Jon's asking what he wanted Elaine to know about him, G replied:

> *How much I have love for her life. I'm not saying that I love her, but I have a strong, strong love for her life.*

Asked what he didn't want to know about Elaine, *G replied:*

> *That someday she will really succeed in killing herself.*

G's response seems to indicate that, to some extent, he had needed not to know that Elaine is dangerously suicidal and possibly psychotic.

Asked what he didn't want Elaine to know about him, G answered:

> *Well, I wouldn't want her to know that I've had some erotic fantasies about her.*

G made it clear that he never had any intention of acting on his fantasies, but that he believed that this was not the time in their treatment to explore sexual feelings and concerns.

Jon then invited G to assume the "you" position and instructed him to "become" Elaine by imitating her facial expressions, gestures, way of speaking, etc., He indicated that he would speak to G as if he were Elaine. After imitating Elaine, G spoke as if he were her by saying;

> *I hate April. There are so many birthdays in the month, and I don't know what to buy people. And I don't want to spend so much money for their birthdays. I hate being sure that they will not be happy with my gifts and that they will be angry with me.*

When the Supervisor asks G (as Elaine) what it was like to tell these things to G, G (as Elaine) answered:

> *I'm not sure I'm talking to G. I feel alone inside—and separate. it's funny I feel as if I'm talking to my father when he doesn't listen to me."*

Here G realizes not only that his sense of feeling disconnected from Elaine is shared by her but that she may have experienced being with him as she has felt with her father.

Jon echoes what G (as Elaine) has said for emphasis:

"*So,* it's like talking to your father when he doesn't listen to you."

G (as Elaine) adds: *"Yes, it's like nobody hears me."*

When asked what she would like to know about G, G (as Elaine) says: *"I don't know. It's like I've lost him. It's like talking to a stranger."*

Asked what she wants G to know about her, G (as Elaine) answers: *"That I'm so lost."*

In response to the question about what she doesn't want to know about G, G (as Elaine) answers; *"I don't know."* The tone of G's voice as he imitated Elaine conveys that she doesn't want any connection to him.

Asked what she doesn't want G to know about her.

G (as Elaine) says: *"That I'm so scared."*

All these responses seem to confirm G's experience that, like him, Elaine has lost all sense of connectedness with him and that there is danger associated with this disruption between them.

When asked to enter the "We" position by forming an image of the relationship between him and Elaine as he imitated her. G says:

> It's funny, both of us are in front of our own fathers and both of us have lost the capacity to talk. We are trapped in our own spaces. We are each sure we will never be listened to or heard. Our fathers are still so strong. They rob of us of what we might build together and create together.

G has come to realize that not only is Elaine fearful that G, like her father, cannot hear her fear that she will kill herself, but also that Elaine's fear of her father has reminded G of his own father who could not listen to him. We believe that in answering the questions related to relational knowing, G became better able to understand what had led him to feel that his connection to his patient had been lost. It was not merely that G had not wanted to know how seriously disturbed his patient was, but by "becoming" Elaine, he felt empty and alone—just as he had felt with his own father. This appears to have been a turning point for him. G expressed relief that on realizing that his own feelings of disconnection from his own father had been reenacted between him and Elaine.

Asked if he wanted to experiment with some new way of being with Elaine, G said, *"I would like to try talking to her almost as if she were the therapist (not that she would really be the therapist) but that I could let her know what had gotten in the way of our relating."*

G now has some hope that by revealing to Elaine that he was triggered by painful memories of being with his unresponsive father, he could possibly repair the major disruption between them.

When the group members were invited to become Elaine's therapists after G imitated her once more, their reactions to G's patient were intense; Here are some example:

> *I felt anger on her behalf. I felt like saying 'I hate your father or fuck him,' or something like that.*
>
> *I felt intense heat in my body as if it were like fire. And then what happened is that I identified completely with her, and I saw myself vomiting in the face of a figure that I thought was the therapist.*

"I just felt very, very sad, like a physical weight of sadness."

> *I felt physically cold and there was a lot of discomfort in my chest. But it also made me want to let go of her. I had this image--I'm holding the rope to Elaine but it's so uncomfortable for me that I have to fight not to just let it go and drift away. I think that I as a therapist would want to almost kind of resign.*

G seemed to find the group's reactions confirming of his own sense that the loss of a sense of connectedness with Elaine was extremely distressing. They also let him get in touch with the difficulties that he might still encounter in regaining his sense of therapeutic competence in working with Elaine.

We now offer a supervisory relationship that was less about feeling that the connection between therapist and patient was lost, but rather that it was too intense.

L and Tina

L explained that his main reason for seeking supervision for his therapeutic relationship with Tina, a severely traumatized 58-year-old woman, was to get help dealing with her urgent need for contact after sessions. During their five-year long relationship, Tina had managed to maintain her employment in a large corporation, but her life outside of work seemed to L to be "crumbling."

To provide some background for his challenging work with Tina, L mentioned that she had been bullied as a child and that her parents had been rejecting, demanding and punishing. In an intensely dissociated state during one session with L, Tina had said, "I can't breathe, my arms are too short and I'm bleeding." In response to L's questions, Tina revealed that she was bleeding from her vagina. She then remembered having been raped repeatedly by a neighbor which started when she was only six years old and lasted several years.

Aside from the wrenching distress Tina exhibited during sessions, L was often greatly upset by Tina's frequent calls to him outside of sessions saying that she felt suicidal and distraught. L also found it difficult to get Tina to leave his office at the end of sessions.

The supervisor (Doris) suggested that L try working in the "I" position. Asked to describe what he felt in his body when he imagined seeing Tina again, L said:

> *I can feel this lump in my belly, I also feel sadness in my chest because her history is like a bad horror movie--so gruesome--so brutal. But it's also difficult not to be somehow angry because she can be really demanding.*

Doris then asked L to "become" Tina by imitating her expressions, gestures, etc. and that she will relate to L as if he were Tina. In response to being asked what L (as Tina) is experiencing? L (as Tina, said: *"I don't know, just chaos. chaos."*

Asked how it felt to be with L, L (as Tina) answered: *"It's safe here. It's very important to be safe. That's so much chaos and nobody cares."*

When asked if L cares about the chaos that you live in, L (as Tina) replied: *"He tries but he is just a professional--even so, it feels safer to be with this professional than not to be here."*

Asked about not wanting to leave the office, L (as Tina) says: "Yeah, it's scary to leave the office. I don't know what to do outside. I just have to run."

L's empathic grasp of Tina's reasons for not wanting to leave sessions and her need to be in contact with him has become increasingly evident to him.

When L was asked to move to the "We" position and to try to form an image of himself and Tina, he replied.

> *Tina is a patient who is quite honest, and she has a great sense of humor, so It's quite scary and entertaining at the same time.*

Doris commented: So, there is something going on that is almost pleasurable about what's happening between the two of you,

L then added: "*I learn quite a bit in working with Tina. I must go very deep to learn more and more. She's having quite a huge influence on me. She can be very demanding, but I learn something new all the time".*

Doris commented: So, she is really bringing out the best in you in a way. She's making you go deeper.

On entering the following Zoom meeting in which he was asked the relational knowing questions, L reported: "I've *been thinking about last session a lot and I think Tina and I have shared so much madness."* L then gave examples of unconventional things he has done during sessions with Tina *such as* banging on a drum when she is lost in a dissociated state to bring her back to the session.

When asked what he would like to know about Tina, L said:

> *I have no idea what I would like to know. It's the opposite. There is so much coming from her that it's more important to have some filters and barriers.*

L's concern about setting limits in his work with Tina is apparent here. When asked what he wanted Tina to know about him, L replied:

> I care. The main theme of our work is to convince her to believe that I actually care about her as a person.

When asked what he didn't want to know about Tina, L said:

> *"Maybe not some concrete facts about her suffering. It's just too much." L added: " And maybe even her emotions. I don't need to know everything. Even on this emotional level, it's just too much."*

Doris notes that she feels that it's important for L to be honest about the limits of his tolerance for the intensity of Tina's suffering.

Asked what he didn't want Tina to know about him, L replied:

> *It's two quite different things. First, since she can be quite intrusive, I don't want her to know too many private things about me; secondly, I don't want her to know the full effect of her demands on me. It would just produce so much self-hate in her.*

Doris then asked the relational knowing questions to L as Tina:

> In response to the question, What do you want to know about L. L (as Tina) answered: *"I would like to really know if he cares or if he pretends because he is professional."*

Asked, "What would you like him to know about you?", L (as Tina) replied, *"There is little he does not know."*

L (as Tina) then replied to the question, "What do you want L not to know about you?": "That I'm so bad, such an ugly person."

And is there something that you don't want to know about L?

> *if he does things because he is just a doctor, then I don't want to know it.*

L has come to deeply appreciate Tina's need to feel that he truly cares for her but that there are limits to his capacity to be there for her. He is not entirely clear about how to set limits but is now in touch with his creativity in working with Tina.

Here are some responses from the group as they tried to become Tina's therapist:

> *I felt like I was watching a horror movie. I got scared. It was like one of those movies with some person who's possessed or something like that. And I got really cold, really, really cold. I felt tired, a bit like this is so much. I feel like I can't contain this. Like this is too much.*

"I had the same feeling--like I'm watching 'The Shining,' watching a character in a horror movie with a feeling of, 'my God, this poor little thing, so scared to be outside.' "

> *I just wanted to say that this week after the time in between that I feel quite affectionate about her and since people were describing that she's so challenging and demanding and can be very difficult, I thought I would just share that the way I feel about her is quite tender.*

L seems to have experienced the groups responses as confirmation that Tina had undergone horrific abuse, that she elicits compassion, and that L's need to set limits on her demands was shared. L realized that while there is gratification for him in working with Tina, he will have to draw on his creativity to find ways to tolerate her intense needs for contact.

In the following examples, we try to show a range of concerns that supervisees had about their therapeutic relationships and how the addition of the embodied relational knowing questions enriched their understanding of their patients and themselves.

D and Hannah

D had started her relationship with Hannah, a severely traumatized woman of 25. Living on her own after the untimely death of her mother and subsequently abandoned by her father, Hannah, still a teenager, moved from the house of one friend to another for many months. She married her first boyfriend when she was only 19.

D described Hannah as very shy, anxious and reticent to speak about her life. She suffers from symptoms of PTSD including recurring thoughts and images related to her mother's final moments. Nevertheless, D described Hannah as resourceful enough to have finished a bachelor's degree.

Asked what she wanted to work on in the supervisory session, D replied that despite Hannah's having formed a close maternal transference with her, she was concerned that the treatment was "stuck." She noted that Hannah can be quite concrete and that she sometimes feels frustrated with her.

In the "**I**" position, D said:

> *I feel my heart beating. This is going to be tough. I'm on edge. What's she going to bring? It's very strange how anxious I'm feeling. Then she added, "Now I feel sad because I feel a little bit like I don't want to let her in. I am on the edge of crying.*

In answer to the question, "What do you want to know about Hannah?" D said, *"First thing that popped in my mind was, 'Is she okay?'"*

Asked what she wanted Hannah to know about her, D said, *"That she's loved—that she's kind of remarkable is the word that keeps going around. And the other thing is she doesn't have to experience herself as small."*

With these answer D seems to have confirmed her concern about Hannah and her positive feelings for her, but when asked what she didn't want to know about Hanna, she answered,

> *That maybe there's something darker or sadder or that she's really not okay. That she's more depleted and blank than I see.*

D seems to have realized that she had not fully allowed herself to consider that Hannah might be more troubled than she had initially assumed.

She added that she didn't want Hannah to know *"that I'm scared I can't help her. That I can't actually do anything for her that's going to really help."*

In the "You" position, D (as Hannah) was asked what she wanted to know about D. D (as Hannah) answered,

> *Nothing. Nothing really. I know a lot.*

With this response D confirmed her sense that the relationship was not at all reciprocal, that Hannah experienced D as a maternal figure.

When asked, "What do you want D to know about you?

D (as Hannah) answered: *"That I'm really lonely. I'm really lonely."*

Asked what she didn't want D to know about her, she said: *"How much I need her and kind of wish she was more here."*

These responses suggest that D was now more in touch with the central dilemma of her work with Hannah. She cared deeply for her but she feared that Nina wanted more of her than she felt able to provide.

Replying to the question about what she didn't want to know about D, D (as Hannah replied).

> *That she doesn't like me or I'm too much work. I think she's nice. I don't want to know anything bad or mean about her.*

Here D seems to have reinforced her awareness of the tension in the relationship around her fear that Hannah needed and possibly require more than she is willing to provide.

Interestingly in the "We" position, the image that occurred to D was of two cats circling one another. After reflecting on this, D added,

> But they're okay. They're kind of existing together and kind of okay.

In the next supervisory session, D reported that her work in the supervision group had allowed her to relax with Hannah, and that she had become less anxious with her. We imagine that what allowed D to feel more comfortable with Hannah was her sense that the care and concern she felt for Hannah was helping and that even if Hanna was more troubled than she imagined she did not have to provide more than she felt she felt able to.

E and Paul

Paul, a teen-age boy had told E that he believed he was a psychopath on account of his lack of feelings. Asked what she wanted to know about Paul, E answered:

> *I want to know where he is in his body and how he got to this question of psychopathy.*

Asked what she wanted Paul to know about her, she said:

"I want Paul to know that I know him." E mentioned that if he did it might help him feel connected to her.

Asked what she doesn't want to know about Paul, she replied:

"Well, that's a hard one. I don't want to know that he's a psychopath." then she added: *"But there's very little, I don't want to know about Paul."*

In response to the question about what she doesn't want Paul to know about her, she said:

> *I don't want him to know that I have had a similar feeling—like I don't belong.*

What E had not realized until this point was her sense of being like her patient insofar as she too had a life-long sense of not belonging.

Assuming the "you" position and imitating Paul, E speaks as Paul by saying:

> *So, I want to talk today about, oh wait, wait, wait, wait. Okay. So, I want to talk today about my grandfather, the husband of the grandmother that died. He's 91 and he's not coherent and I don't like how he's acting. It makes me very uncomfortable, but I can't really feel that. So, I think I'm a psychopath.*

The supervisor addressed E as if he were talking to Paul.

"I see. Okay. Paul, how is it for you to tell this to E?"

E (as Paul) answers:

> *Well, it's a little strange, but I know her so long, so I know she's going to know if I am or not* (a psychopath) *and she's going to tell me why, but she may not want to believe me. That's the problem.*

Until this point G had not realized that Paul understood that she was struggling with knowing if he really was a psychopath.
Supervisor:

> Paul, what do you want to know about your therapist?

E (as Paul) answers:

> *I think I want to know if she's ever felt like this.*

E's response indicates her awareness that her patient longed to feel that he was not alone with his doubts and fears and that he would feel less alone if his therapist had also felt painful doubts about herself.
Supervisor asks:

> And what do you want E to know about you?

E (as Paul) answers:

> *Well, I hide, so I want her to get through.*
> *Get through to my . . . I hide.*

E had confirmed her own hunch that Paul wanted her to see behind his deceptions.
Supervisor:

> I see. And what don't you want to know about E?

E (as Paul) answers:

> *That's interesting. Well, I guess I wouldn't want to know that she too was a psychopath.*

E now appreciated that for Paul, being a psychopath (which seems to relate to not having feelings) is a horrible condition that he truly fears.

Supervisor:

And lastly, what don't you want E to know about you?

E (as Paul) answers:

> *That I'm damaged.*

When asked to form an image of their interaction, E replies:

> *It's a tug of war now. I feel like it's a tug of war. I get very persistent about having to persuade him that he is feeling so intensely that it scares him. But Paul refuses to accept it. And so that tug of war keeps going back and forth.*

Asked how she thinks the dialogue is developing, E remarks:

> It's going slowly. She adds that she needs patience and that she cares very much for Paul. She expressed concern about Paul's denial of his feelings and wonders if he might be pretending that he doesn't feel.

By the end of the supervisory session, E realized that what she most needed to know about her relationship with Paul was not if he really was a psychopath but how to address his sense that he was not able to feel his emotions and that he was "damaged." She also learned that she had many uncertainties about how to proceed with Paul. Should she reveal that she too experienced a sense of not belonging in her life? Would that be relieving or concerning to Paul? What might she do to "get through" to him when he so strongly denied his feelings? How should she address his sense of being "damaged?'

Although E felt clearer about what had created the sense of a "tug of war" between her and Paul, she realized that she needed patience and more time to resolve their conflicts. Yet, she believed that her good feelings for Paul would allow her to find increasingly sensitive ways to help him.

T and Christian

After giving a brief introductory account of his relationship with a suicidal man who had injured his own child, T was asked to report on what he experienced in his body in the "I" position. T replied, *"I feel like grinding my teeth. I feel heavy, very heavy."* T could not put into words what was causing his anxious, depressed bodily experience. Asked what he wanted to know about Christian, he said, *"I want to know what it felt like for him to hurt his child."* T simply had not been able to imagine what this man, whom he had grown to like immensely could have experienced while injuring his child. T wondered if he had reached the limit of his empathic ability in relating to Christian.

Asked what he wanted Christian to know about him, he said, *"That he can trust me. That I can have sympathy for him even though I'm horrified by what he did."* When asked the final question: "What didn't he want his patient to know about him," his answer was dramatic and revealing. T said: "That part of me thinks he should have killed himself."

Because T had not been aware of feeling that this man should have killed himself, the supervisory exercise allowed him to feel more compassion for himself. He now appreciated the intensity of his struggle to open his heart to his patient, a man he genuinely cared for, despite his horror at the patient's actions. More in touch with his own complicated reactions he was able to become more interested in what had led to his patient's abusive behavior.

Summary

Perhaps the very act of participating in a supervisory session involves the therapists' acknowledgment of not completely knowing their patients, themselves in relation to their patients, and the best way to help their patients. Yet we can think of no way to help therapists gain confidence in the healing potential of their heir work than through supervision. We believe that with the addition of the embodied relational knowing questions supervisees are helped to gain access to ways of exploring the therapeutic relationship that points them toward deeper and increasingly complex ways to engage in healing.

Reference

Brothers, D. & Sletvold, J. (2023). Talking Bodies: A New Vision of Psychoanalysis. *Psychoanalytic Inquiry*, 42(4): 289–302. https://doi.org/10.1080/07351690.2022.2059292

10 Knowing World

Applauding a dialogue between Orna Guralnik, an Israeli analyst who leads the docuseries, "Couples Therapy," and Christine Harb, a Palestinian-American participant in the series, (Benjamin, 2025) observes:

> (Their dialogue could) enlighten us about what psychoanalytic process in contexts of mass trauma and political difference can aspire to when partners in dialogue commit to intense honesty and the determination to be known by the Other as well as knowing them.
>
> (Benjamin, 2025, pp. 78–82, parenthesis added)

We would say that being known and knowing others is not merely what the psychoanalytic process aspires to—these needs lie at the heart of psychoanalysis. They become particularly urgent in the context of horrific world events such as the bloody conflict that so long endured between Israelis and Palestinians living in Gaza and the West Bank.

Even if no deadly crisis were roiling our world, it might still be true that the more deeply we believe that we know others and feel that they know us just as well, the less vulnerable we feel to the threat of attacks—both physical and psychological—and better able to withstand experiences of life's inescapable uncertainty. But especially during times of dire world conflicts our going-on-being (Winnicott, 1965) as a community of humans seems to depend upon our experiencing a sense of connectedness to others that cannot be sustained in the absence of this sort of knowing.

The need not to know or be known seems to be just as urgent as the need to know or be known in these contexts. In Chapter 2 we tried to demonstrate that the need not to know goes beyond traumatic experiences and is pervasive in everyday life. Needing not to know about the world seems to have intensified in our era. In a commentary in the Norwegian newspaper, Klassekampen, the commentator, Olav Elgvin (2025) noted that in recent years psychologists and social researchers have found that we humans often choose the path of "willful ignorance" or "deliberate ignorance" about events that make us

DOI: 10.4324/9781003487883-11

uncomfortable—particularly when knowing would compromise our sense of ourselves as "good."

Yet we are not convinced that we are ever completely ignorant about how the leaders of a country have chosen to inflict pain and suffering on the vulnerable, or that they are restricting our freedom, or that they are immoral and corrupt. Do we really not know that our lifestyles contribute to the destruction of the earth? That we do not help those in need despite our ability to do so? And that we are biased in favor of those who share our race, ethnicity and social class? Do the leaders themselves really not know the harm they are inflicting? Do they believe the lies they tell?

We suspect that when it comes to world matters, we are often caught in a strange state of both knowing and not knowing. In Chapter 3 we discussed the ways in which dreams intersect both knowing and not knowing and that what had been disguised and hidden in the dream narrative may come to light in the psychoanalytic encounter. We believe that at times of societal upheaval the needs to know and not know merge in a kind of dream state that allows us to keep living as if nothing had changed. Yet our obliviousness may set the stage for our worst nightmares. it seems that what is disguised in ordinary dreams may take the form of silence or lies—or both—in the context of world events.

Dori Laub and Nanette Auerhahn, who have researched methods for helping survivors of societal traumas give testimony, understand this phenomenon from their own perspective. They write:

> We all hover at different distances between knowing and not knowing about trauma, caught between the compulsion to complete the process of knowing and the inability or fear of doing so. It is the nature of trauma to elude our knowledge, because of both defense and deficit. The knowledge of trauma is fiercely defended against, for it can be a momentous, threatening, cognitive and affective task, involving an unjaundiced appraisal of events and our own injuries, failures, conflicts and losses.
>
> (Laub & Auerhahn, 1993, p. 28)

Our ideas about the merger of needing to know and not know borrow extensively from the writings of Roger Frie (2017, 2020) who discussed this phenomenon with respect to his discovery that his beloved grandfather had been a member of the NSKK or National Socialist Motor Corps, a paramilitary organization of the Nazi party in Germany during World War II.

Frie (2020) writes:

> What does it mean to be confronted with an unspoken history, to be caught in a web of the past over which we have no control? We are each born into a history and culture that precedes us. At some point in our lives we may be able to reflect on the historical narratives we inherit and

> begin to question them. At other moments we may encounter powerful counternarratives that demonstrate the limits of what we assume to be true.
>
> (Frie, 2020, p. 6)

In her discussion of a previous paper by Frie written in 2019, Sue Grand (2019) notes that we all share "Frie's ethical/familial/cultural predicament." Acknowledging the complexity of Frie's moral position she asks:

> What will we allow ourselves to see and to know? Where do we find ethical agency and an empowered responsibility? Will we sacrifice the Other to deny our fear and shame? How is this moment reflecting all of our transgenerational ghosts: the victims, bystanders, and perpetrators of our own history? Can inherited guilt and shame become generative forces? Finally, that hardest of ethical questions: Is there a difference between our ordinary human badness and a radical evil that cannot, and should not, be humanized? Is there hope of a humanizing discourse with the alt-right? Can we come to know, and ameliorate, such hate and violence?
>
> (Grand, 2019, p. 148)

Given the enormity of what we believe is at stake, the answers given to Grand's questions are crucially important for our patients and ourselves. Yet, the convergence of the need to know and the need not to know may make for confusing analytic encounters. The analytic partners may not attend to references about the horrors on the world stage that are hidden or disguised in rather banal conversations. Our clinical examples of analytic hatred in Chapter 5 probably reflect, to some extent, our failure to detect the influence of the world on what was going on between us and our patients. We suspect that Jon's patient both needed to know and not to know Jon's political affiliations. It is also likely that both Doris and her patient both knew how destructively competitive the publishing world can be. More importantly, they both knew and didn't know how envy and power in that world had influenced their feelings about one another.

Stories about the collisions of the need to know and not know with respect to political situations can be found in recent newspaper accounts. For example, in a May 16th 2025 opinion piece in the New York Times, entitled, "How Did So Many Elected Democrats Miss Biden's Infirmity?", Michelle Goldberg writes that even after she had written a column arguing that Biden was too old to run for a second term, some officials and pundits mentioned that Biden's legislative successes proved he was still up to the job. She writes:

> "Some of them seemed so sure I was mistaken that I wondered if they might be right." Commenting on a book by Jake Tapper and Alex Thomson's book, "Original Sin", exposing Biden's deterioration, Goldberg writes: ". . . more than lying to the public about Biden's increasing infirmity, I think too many Democrats were lying to themselves."

Goldberg attributes the coverup of Biden's infirmity to the fact that "gerontocracy" is increasingly the norm in American politics. While her assertion may be true, we suspect that in this instance, the need not to know outweighed the need to know for those close to Biden. They certainly both needed to know and needed not to know what the alternative to his being elected might be.

Many of our patients have mentioned needing not to hear about the destructive forces that are ravaging the world. They mention having stopped listening to news programs on television and on their phones. In effect, they prefer silence. Silence, we believe, goes a long way towards allowing for the merger of knowing and not knowing. We know, for example, that we are doomed to die, but we rarely speak of our deaths. Perhaps not mentioning death allows us to maintain a fantasy that we will live forever. Silence also frequently surrounds death by suicide. Not speaking may help us avoid painful feelings of shame and guilt for failing to have kept a lost loved one alive.

Consider how Thato Letsatsi (2025) writes about silence in her effort to explore racial trauma:

> Silence can be experienced as both a mask and a mirror—hiding what we fear to name while revealing emotional truths that are previously unknown or that we are not ready to face. It can shield us from experiences of vulnerability or offer solace and reverence when words feel too fragile. Sometimes it can be experienced as a wound; at other times, as a wall. It may hold guilt, grief, overwhelm, or unspoken longing. Silence can punish, protect, or transform, if we show up and stay present in its tension and dialogue with it.
>
> Letsatsi (2025)

Similarly, Frie (2020) notes:

> There are different kinds of silence and silencing at work. . . it is the silence of perpetrators and enablers that leads to the silencing of victims. Societies that have something to be ashamed of frequently silence those who might wish to speak out. The silence of the present reinforces the silencing of the past. Silence and silencing shapes what it said and not said, which voices are heard, and whether we are willing to listen.
>
> (Frie, 2020, p. 7)

We have found that silence follows many societal disasters. Doris remembers asking an audience at a trauma conference in South Africa soon after the end of Apartheid about their experiences of the traumas during this period. She was met with absolute silence. First responders in the aftermath of the September 11th 2001 attacks on the World Trade Center in New York, refused to talk about their experiences for many months (Goren, 2011).

Many patients seem unable to break their silence with words about traumatic experiences until much time has passed. It is not that they do not know that the traumas occurred; they simply do not anticipate being able to bear the feelings this knowing will arouse. With the establishment of safe, trusting analytic relationships that demonstrate that feelings do become more bearable when they are heard without judgment, the words come more easily.

But patients are not the only ones who must be helped to speak of the painful conflicts that reverberate throughout this traumatized and traumatizing world; we therapists must also be helped to end our silence. What stops us from speaking of the horrors that, like slow moving rivers of lava, seem destined to smother all that is vital, beautiful and joyful in our lives? What keeps us from helping one another find ways to have conversations about clashing political perspectives and the racial, class, sex and gender struggles that are fracturing our world?

We suspect that what enters our analytic relationships from the world is not a one-way street and that what happens in our consulting rooms does affect what happens outside our closed doors. Letsatsi notes that when she presented her views on racial trauma, she could feel anxiety—both her own and that of the audience, but that when the discussion opened, the shared anxiety was transformed. Perhaps patients who feel some degree of healing after giving voice to their painful relational conflicts make a difference in the world. Max Sucharov (personal communication) uses complexity theory to understand this possibility. He notes that "No utterance, text, paper, book is created by an isolated author but is an emergent property of the open human system. The relative contribution of various individuals is *in principle* indeterminate." He characterizes this idea as "quantum relational holism."

Without naively believing in a single potent psychoanalytic method guaranteed to produce sudden and complete change, we have discovered a number of contemporary analysts whose work seems to point us toward lessening the need not to know and helping us find ways to end silence. We now offer a few examples of statements and writings by psychoanalytic thinkers that we believe help to break the silence.

Let us begin with words by Donna Orange (2022) on the devastation of our ongoing climate emergency that appear in her article entitled, "Climate justice and Radical Ethics":

What is climate justice? Like every justice discourse, it means acknowledging and addressing injustice. It includes the psychoanalytic work of remembering (colonization, chattel slavery, and their lived continuance today) and working through. Working through includes the work of repentance, repair and reparation.

> Today we live in a war-ravaged world sustained in its injustice and violence by an international commitment to oil, gas, and coal. These are creating temperature rises at rates historically unknown, sea level rise, polar melting, desertification, rapid destruction of irreplaceable species, long and terrifying fire seasons, and forms of extreme weather we had never seen. Those who suffer most from the climate emergency are those who

> have contributed to it the least, our brothers and sisters from Latin America, Africa, and the middle East. Remembering what is happening, why it is happening, and the extreme injustice of what is happening is psychoanalytic work, whether we call it that or not. Remembering that at least half the greenhouse gases destroying our home planet have come during the past 25 years means we who are alive today have committed this creeping crime against humanity.
>
> (Orange, 2022, p. 339)

She adds her plea to psychoanalysts to provide help for the young activists whom she says, need our voices and our bodies.

> Even if we cannot join them on hunger strikes, we can teach our colleagues, our children and our grandchildren that climate emergency also means devastation for our hungry and homeless sisters and brothers around the world. We can walk or bicycle instead of driving or flying, as often as possible. We can stop buying "stuff" made by horribly underpaid workers and shipped to us at tremendous climate cost.
>
> (Orange, 2022, p. 339)

Another plea to analysts was made by Max Sucharov in his 2022 article entitled, "The Ugly Truth to Canada's Big Lie: A Tale of Ongoing Settler Colonial Genocide of Canada's Indigenous Peoples and the Creation of an Apartheid State." In his "final comments," Sucharov writes:

> My principal goal in writing this paper is to raise awareness to both myself and my non-indigenous colleagues, especially my Canadian settler colleagues. My hope is that my settler colleagues will conduct their own inquiry and confirm for themselves the deplorable reality of ongoing genocidal racism against Canada's Indigenous peoples.
>
> (Sucharov, 2022, p. 205)

He then challenges us to act:

> Find about more about the Indian Act. Find out more about the reserve system. To my Indigenous readers, please let me know of any evidence of conscious or unconscious "settler pullback" by my possible minimizing or whitewashing historical and/or contemporary Indigenous suffering at the hands of Canada's colonial government or by racist individuals. Writing of this paper has constituted a sometimes painful and humbling learning experience . . . Even though my eyes have been open for only a brief portion of my 76 years, this journal issue does not have enough space to record all I have witnessed of traumatizing and genocidal racism against Indigenous peoples living in what is now called Canada.
>
> (Sucharov, 2022, p. 205)

Ilene Philipson calls our attention to the ways in which the recent turn in psychoanalysis toward the social and political have affected analytic institutions. She began a presentation at the 2025 IAPSP conference in Pasadena by wondering if analysts today have lost the love of psychoanalysis that was apparent in the outpouring of emotion that she witnessed for Heinz Kohut who was near death when he gave his final talk in 1981.

While acknowledging the benefits of the current focus on society and politics insofar as it has made it more likely that we analysts consider our own socially constructed biases, she notes that rather than using our empathy and curiosity to understand the social, "we have replicated and promoted the vitriol, binary thinking, moralism, and certitude that dominate our current, political landscape." She suggests that displacement has come to serve as a means of expressing agency and empowerment absent for us in the larger political arena. She writes:

> Attacking other analysts, our institutes, and organizations for being racist, transphobic, and/or antisemitic may emerge from honest concerns about injustice. But frequently such concerns are expressed with unmetabolized affect, condemnation rather than discussion.

She also describes the enormous task we face:

> Our challenge remains the ability to acknowledge our anxieties, our grief, and our outrage about the direction our societies are moving and not displace those feelings onto other analysts and our institutes and organizations. Can we use the insights provided by our theories and apply them to understanding the society in which we live, to use psychoanalysis to interrogate authoritarianism, rather than mimicking the rancor, rage, and certitude that characterizes the authoritarian states of mind we see in society at large?

Sue Grand offers an insightful and inspiring understanding of the consequences of silence and blindness. She writes:

> The authors exhort us to bring our private, relational bodies into an ethical knowing of the social world. This social world seems split between the architects of greed and power, and the brutalized Other who starves at the oligarch's behest. How much do we want to know of this Other? What are the consequences of our silence and blindness? For the authors, there is a perpetual tension between knowing and not-knowing. This tension may be most acute in those reckoning with trauma. As the authors note, the paradox of knowing-not-knowing has many meanings and functions in the aftermath of trauma. Some of these functions are life and world sustaining. However, if we look at human history, our not-knowing is clearly the devil's playground. The tension between looking and not-looking, between

> blindness and perception: as I have suggested (see Grand, 2000), this creates a paralytic psycho-social field where destructiveness is ascendant. In this "malignant dissociative contagion" (Grand, 2000), we each hold multiple positions, alternately resisting, and obscuring, violence. The forces of domination are invested in this obscurity. When we are not looking, destructiveness "moves fast and breaks things". Justice moves slower; and justice delayed is justice denied.
>
> This paralytic social field, this tendency towards silence and blindness, this perpetual iteration of violence: this looks endemic to our "normative" human condition. Maybe Freud was right about Thanatos. Maybe greed and hatred are just more elemental, more compelling, than human kindness. If so, we are doomed by the world destroying forces around us. We cannot accept this framing of our "normative" human condition. Instead, we need to query it. In my own work, I have been focused on the trans-generational transmission of our perpetrator parts. As these authors suggest, we want to know ourselves as good. The most deeply dissociated aspect of our trans-generational heritage is our own persecutory legacy. We refuse to know ourselves, and our loved ones, as agents of destruction. We are always, and only, victims. I, me, us: we were never persecutory. But in that refusal, we split off our own turn towards violence, project it into the Other, renew ourselves as innocent victims, and legitimize our own greed and aggression as "justice". We cannot stop the cycle of violence without knowing that we, ourselves, are agents of harm. If we fully bring our intimate, knowing, relational bodies into dialogue with the persecuted Other, Eros may triumph over Thanatos.

In a talk entitled, "Keeping a Multilayered Perspective in a Troubled World that he presented at the 2025 IAPSP conference in Pasadena, Haim Weinberg addressed what he characterized as "the challenges of maintaining a non-binary perspective on social and political processes in today's world." After suggesting ways in which Heinz Kohut's constructs of empathy, mirroring and idealization might apply to organizational cultures, group processes and political life, and discussing his group analytic perspective, Weinberg advanced his ideas about using a large group model to overcome social ruptures.

He explains:

> In Large Groups, people can examine their relationship to authority figures, attraction to charismatic leaders, witness scapegoating and disavowal of the unwanted parts of the self, as well as civility, finding one's voice, and a sense of connection derived from camaraderie and belonging. The LG focus is on transpersonal issues beyond the personal and the interpersonal, with consideration given to unconscious social processes. What cannot be discussed (is dissociated, repressed, or disavowed) in public discourse is

> enacted in society. The LG, when convened well, provides a safe place to discuss these unspoken social topics. events, and their own participation in systemic racism and bias.
>
> If the LG process is successful, members learn a different way of communicating about divisive social issues, moving from a binary debate (in which each side brings the best arguments to convince the other that they hold the absolute truth) to a dialogue (in which each party is curious about the point of view of the other). However, since the safety of a supportive, well-contained small group is absent in the LG, our model integrates LG and SG meetings, which deepens the exploration of personal insights and meanings found in the LG.

Weinberg presents an illustration of a group that had been meeting for several years that included 10 therapists from a variety of countries. He describes how a question, "Who here is a Zionist," aroused tensions and withdrawal. He attempted to redirect the conversation from political argument to emotional experience. Examining his own countertransference, he asked to be held accountable if a group member sensed bias, given his identity as a Jew. He then describes how the group shifted and that a final session ended with a sense of relief and reconciliation.

Weinberg explains:

> What allowed this positive outcome? I believe that transparency about my positionality, emphasis on dialogue over debate, and explicit permission for members to hold me accountable were key. Yet the process was messy, slow, and imperfect—much like real life.

Stacy Berlin offers suggestions about how analysts might engage in dialogues about gender and sexuality. She writes:

> How do we break the silence surrounding the conflicts over sex and gender unfolding across the globe today? How do we create conditions for dialogue rather than division? The tension between witnessing and withdrawal, splitting and holding, speaking and silence, is not new. Yet this moment returns us to psychoanalysis's ethical roots: to listen not only to the individual but also to the social and political forces that shape psychic life, and to the ways these forces live between analyst and patient. Silence can preserve safety, but it can also calcify into complicity when harm and exclusion go unnamed. To speak, then, is to extend psychoanalysis's reach, to articulate suffering and transformation in a way that is neither didactic nor moralizing but attuned to the unconscious tides that may either deaden or enliven our collective life. As Bromberg (1998) reminds us, vitality emerges when we can "stand in the spaces" between positions without collapsing them, when we allow multiplicity and contradiction to coexist without premature synthesis. As Gaztambide (2019) argues, psychoanalysis at its

> most alive is an act of radical love: a decolonial practice that faces power and difference without retreating into neutrality or moral superiority. Love, in this sense, is both political and ethical, insists on our shared vulnerability and interdependence, even when it exposes our complicity. This love resonates with Benjamin's (1988) notion of mutual recognition, the fragile capacity to see and be seen as subjects without negating the other's separateness. For Benjamin, recognition is precarious and easily lost, yet it remains the precondition for ethical relatedness.
>
> The analytic dyad becomes a microcosm of the world's fractures, where social asymmetries, what Layton (2010) calls the "social unconscious" of privilege and marginalization, are replayed in enactments, silences, and misrecognitions. To break the silence is to listen to what is enacted and disavowed between us, to tolerate uncertainty and discomfort, and to recognize the moments when our theoretical allegiances obscure more than they reveal. We need not take a political stance in the conventional sense. Rather, we must reclaim psychoanalysis as a practice that acknowledges, as Gaztambide insists, that "the psyche is never untouched by history." Bearing witness does not resolve suffering; it places us in relation to it, holding contradiction and ambivalence. In Ogden's (1994) terms, this means inhabiting the "analytic third," the intersubjective field where both analyst and analysand are transformed by what emerges between them. Creating analytic, communal, and intellectual spaces where such tensions can be thought rather than foreclosed is itself a form of resistance, to polarization, moral certainty, and the disavowal of complexity. Finally, like religion, psychoanalysis cannot expect people to change their minds, but it can help them feel seen. In a climate where the capacity to feel one's own vulnerability, and to see the other without diminishing their worth, has grown rare, our task is to cultivate presence. To engage analysts and our institutions in confronting difference and its discontents is to honor our calling: to break silence not with certainty but with witnessing, humility, and, as Gaztambide might say, with a radical and reparative love, one that remembers that beneath all our conflicts, we are more alike than different.

Lynne Jacobs, who has called analysts' attention to what she describes as "white privilege," discusses the ways in which knowing and not knowing play a role in "human zoos" which were popularized by European and white American cultures in the early 1900s. She writes:

> Remnants of human zoos exist to this day, as Jade E. Davis points out, in her book, *The Other Side of Empathy*. For those who have not been exposed to human zoos, these days they exist as "cultural enactments." For instance, when you tour an unfamiliar country, or an exhibition comes to your country, you may see an exhibit in which local "actors" can be seen

> using farm tools from the past, using a loom for weaving garments of old, etc. The scene is presented as if to show you the roots of a culture that was long ago disavowed or destroyed, and you can look at it with nostalgia, or with appreciation for "their" olden days, while vaguely sensing that you are complicit in the loss that is being enacted. The original human zoos usually contained animals as well as people, and many of the animals and people died from the varying effects of the dislocation they suffered. It is in such moments that you might have a disquieting encounter with your wish to turn away, not from the "zoo," which you might recoil from viscerally, but from your realization of the vastness of all that you ordinarily choose to ignore.

She adds:

> Our imperfect antidote for this problem is simply to gently hold this encounter with our wish to turn away. If we become kind and friendly towards our humility, we can hold this conflict with more grace, more willingness.

We now turn to Daniel Goldin's understanding of what he calls "pragmatic psychoanalysis," an approach that emphasizes the impossibility of excluding the world from our therapeutic relationships.

After noting that "It is hard to square our current focus on the intrapsychic and the intersubjective with happenings outside the room that so obviously drive our thoughts and feelings," Goldin focuses our attention on Fanon. Half a century ago, Goldin notes, "Fanon noted this gap in our theories when he urged a move from an "individual psychology" a la Freud to one that considers what he calls 'sociogeny.' For Fanon, his problems could not be placed squarely in the mind nor in the family (he was raised in Antilles as though white) but outside in a sick myth. It is only 'at the first white gaze,' he writes, "that the black man feels the weight of his melanin."

Goldin then writes:

> Analysts are thus often enjoined to bring up the culture of the patient and the culture of the analyst as an important part of a discourse of difference. The theorist simply appends to an essentially intrapsychic or intersubjective account the fact that a patient is Jewish or black, etc. The problem is that no one is Jewish or black in the abstract. One identifies as Jewish or black, or has that identity forced on one, in particular ways that reach into one's history and involve all one's current circumstances.

Goldin goes on to describe pragmatic psychoanalysis as an alternative:

> I use the word "pragmatic" in three ways. First, I draw from the American philosophical traditions associated with James, Dewey, Peirce and Mead,

> so-called pragmatic philosophy. Pragmatic philosophy, broadly speaking, describes knowing a person as inseparable from knowing how they act within their life-worlds. In other words, a pragmatic psychoanalysis is committed to foregrounding a person's actual lived experience in the culturally saturated world they live in now. Second, relatedly, the work done under the auspices of pragmatic psychoanalysis must be clearly useful to the other person in their current world. Thirdly, Psychoanalysis is understood as a pragmatic enterprise in and of itself. That is to say it is a practice, rather than a theory, that can best be understood in the particular context of particular interactions.

Goldin concludes:

> A pragmatic psychoanalysis offers a more intuitive way to understand culture by keeping the primary focus on the patient's experience outside the room. Culture is not extraneous to this experience. It permeates it.
>
> For the pragmatic psychoanalyst, mind and thought and emotion are never understood as residing inside a person but are always understood as emerging in experience and by extension in the societies where experience takes shape. In the place of concern with the other's "mental health," or concern with levels of relational freedom in the dyad, we put concern with the other's fittedness in their world. This means the world itself is as subject to analysis as the person's history and plans within it.
>
> In working with patients in an empathic way that looks to fittedness between patient and world, we may find ourselves sharing a space of critique, one that is unique to the other person's situation but may also point to a problem shared by many others. We harbor no revolutionary or Utopian ideals, but in our willingness to inhabit a space of critique, we bring a social justice mentality to our work. Pragmatic psychoanalysis is fashioned to be easily imported into community therapy. The hope is that there it might generate a new ethos and many distributed points of light.

The contributions we have included in this chapter address some of the many ways in which we analysts could respond to the harrowing times in which our therapeutic relationships now take place. Many others analytic writers whom we have not referenced in these pages have taken up this challenge as well. Although we cannot hope to match the eloquence of their voices, we hope that by asking questions about the world that correspond to the various aspects of embodied relational knowing we may also help to some extent. We suggest considering the following questions: What do you want to know about the world? What do you not want to know about the world? What do you want the world to know about you? What do you not want the world to know about you? What do you suspect you both want to know and not know?

We end the chapter with the striking answers Mark Freeman, a philosopher and psychologist, has given to our questions.

What Do You Want to Know About the World?

There is a lot I want to know about the world! For present purposes, though, I will limit my response mainly to what's going on politically and culturally in the United States. At a most basic level, I want to know how and why so many people remain under the sway of an ignorant, corrupt, morally repugnant administration. I do, of course, realize that reasons can be adduced: people thought DJT was acting on their behalf or they are single issue (e.g. anti-abortion) people or that they fear their precious country being taken over by Others (etc., etc.), but I still find myself mystified by much of what's going on—and continues to go on. Taking this question to another level, I also want to know who and what we are as a species. In the end, are we fundamentally self-interested, such that when forces come along that allow us *not* to care we jump on the opportunity? Or is it that our care can be so thoroughly overwhelmed and nullified by nefarious forces that we readily succumb to them? Needless to say, there's much more that might be said about all this.

What Do You Not Want to Know About the World

These days, I find myself not wanting to know about the latest bit of sleaze or corruptness or meanness. In some ways, I both want to know and don't want to know (which I know I need to address in response to another question). But the "don't want to know" is often winning out. I don't want to know about DJT's and Jeffrey Epstein's relationship. I don't want to know about Kash Patel's girlfriend. Or Karoline Leavitt's latest pathetic rhetorical twist. It's often just too much, and it leaves me feeling dirty and undernourished by what is good, true, and beautiful. Actually, it's not that I don't want to know about all this stuff; it's that I already do, and it's depleting and demoralizing. Here too, of course, there's much more that might be said.

What Do You Want the World to Know About You?

Hmmm. . . . For present purposes, again, I want the world to know that I care deeply about what's going on and that I'm doing what I can, as a scholar and intellectual (and citizen), to speak to it in some way. This doesn't mean that I feel like I'm doing enough. I could be taking a much more activist stance in relation to some of the issues I care about, and I could be taking more of a leadership role in speaking to these issues. Most important, in any case, is that I want the world to know that I and many of my colleagues are not just locked up in the ivory tower blissfully removed from the challenges the wider world presents but are taking our moral and ethical responsibilities seriously. What exactly does this mean? I'm still trying to figure it out!

What Do You Not Want the World to Know About You?

Where do I begin?! I don't want the world to know that I'm sometimes lazy and unmotivated, that I spent lots of time scrolling through my iPhone and watching cheap tv, that I spend a good deal of time and money on frivolities even while knowing full well that I could be doing otherwise, that I continue to eat meat even though I know it's unhealthy and bad for the environment (and involves killing innocent sentient beings!), that I drink too much even though I know I shouldn't, that even though I think and write a lot about "the priority of the Other," I oftentimes don't live that priority, that I sometimes wonder whether what I do is truly significant (and on and on and on). You get the idea!

What Are the Things You Suspect You Both Want to Know and Not Want to Know?

There are so many different ways of answering this question. For simplicity's sake, I'll just speak of one basic constellation of knowing and not knowing—namely, the atrocities that litter the world: Israel/Gaza, Russia/Ukraine, Sudan, starving children (among others) all over the world, relentless poverty, poor sanitary conditions, the climate crisis (and on and on and on). Of course I don't want to turn my back on all this—and I don't. Nor, though, do I always want to do a deep dive into the latest article detailing the latest horror. (I sometimes turn the page.) So yes, I want to know the full measure of our misery and fallenness as a species. And no, I don't!

References

Benjamin, J. (1988). *The Bonds of Love: Psychoanalysis, Feminism, and the Problem of Domination*. New York: Pantheon.

Benjamin, J. (2025). Dialogues, 35(1): 78–82.

Bromberg, P. M. (1998). *Standing in the Spaces: Essays on Clinical Process, Trauma and Dissociation*. Hillside, N.J.: Analytics Press.

Frie, R. (2019). Hostory's Ethical Demand: Memory, Denial, and Resposibility in the Wake of the Holocaust. *Psychoanalytic Dialogues*, 29: 2.

Frie, R. (2020). Facing the Nazi Past: Silence, Memory and Inhabiting Responsibility. *Psychoanalysis, Self and Context*, 15(1): 5–9.

Gaztambide, D. J. (2019). *A People's History of Psychoanalysis: From Freud to Liberation Psychology*. Lanham, MD: Lexington Books.

Goren, E. (2011). *Beyond the Reach of Ladders*. London: Open Gate Press.

Grand, S. (2000). *The Reproduction of Evil: A Clinical and Cultural Perspective*. New York and London: Routledge.

Grand, S. (2019). Excitations of Vengeance: The We-Ness of History. *Psychoanalytic Dialogues*, 29(2): 143–150. https://doi.org/10.1080/10481885.2019.1587990

Laub. D. & Auerhahn, N. C. (1993). Knowing and Not Knowing Massive Psychic Trauma. *Journal of Psycho-Analysis*, 74: 287–302.

Layton, L. (2010). Irrational Exuberance. Neoliberal Subjectivity and the Perversion of Truth. *Subjectivity*, 3(3): 303–322.

Letsatsi, T. (2025). Intersubjective Taboos: Finding the Other Within. Paper presented at a plenary session of the 46th Annual IAPSP Conference, Pasadena, Ca. October 19, 2025.

Ogen, T.H. (1994). The Analytic Third: Working with Intersubjective Clinical Facts. *International Journal of Psycho-Analysis*, 75: 3–19.

Orange, D. (2022). Radical Ethics in Time of Plague. *Psychoanaltic Inquiry*, 42(2): 113–123

Sucharov, M. (2022). The Ugly Truth to Canada's Big Lie: A Tale of Ongoing Settler Colonial Genocide of Canada's Indigenous Peoples and the Creation of an Apartheid State. *Psychoanalysis, Self and Context,* 17(2): 196–206. https://doi.org/10.1080/24720038.2022.2046753

Weinberg, H. (2025). Keeping a Multilayered Perspective in a Troubled World. Paper presented at a plenary session of the 46th Annual IAPSP Conference, Pasadena, Ca. October 17, 2025.

Winnicott, D. W. (1965). The Maturational Processes and the Facilitating Environment: Studies in the Theory of Emotional Development. International Universities Press.

11 Beyond Knowing

Up to this point, our book describes what we have learned about the complexly interacting needs that constitute embodied relational knowing; the need to know, the need to be known, and the needs not to know or be known. If, as we believe, all knowing is relational—that is, if everything we know stems from our connections to others past and present—not being able to know plunges us into the desolate realm of lonely uncertainty. It is just this forbidding place that we explore in what follows.

Not being able to know about knowing, or anything that involves human relationships for that matter, may be particularly difficult for those of us who have chosen to work in the fields of human psychology. After all, we are in the business of knowing our patients and ourselves. Our efforts to communicate what we know is limited insofar as a great deal of knowing is expressed between "talking bodies," knowledge that lies beyond what we can say with words (Brothers & Sletvold, 2023). Yet there are countless things our bodies cannot tell us. Our effort to learn the intricacies of our embodied vocabularies is very much a work in progress, our knowledge of embodied grammar (the conventions that govern bodily expression) is still rudimentary, and much is lost in translation to the verbal.

Nor can we ever know for certain if what we believe we remember actually happened. Perhaps, as André Aciman (2021, p. 60) puts it: "We remember best what never happened." When we enter the realm that we have described in earlier chapters, in which our need to know collides with our need not to know, fantasy and imagination are likely to complicate our recollections. We certainly have no sure way of knowing what will happen in the future either, even in the next moment.

Think of all that it is impossible to know when we meet new patients. We have no way to predict whether the way their bodies talk to ours in the first meeting will be the same in the next. We have had patients who appeared to be relatively cheerful and optimistic in the initial encounter but seem to have been replaced by despairing, suicidal copies of themselves by the second or third meeting. Did their bodies initially communicate their need not to have

DOI: 10.4324/9781003487883-12

their despair known or were we deaf to the hidden bodily messages of pain and sorrow that were delivered?

Many unanswered questions about the future swirl around a first meeting. Will we eventually grow to love—or hate—the new patient? What power dynamics will emerge? Will this relationship change our lives? And if it does, in what way will it change? How will the relationship end? But there are just as many perplexing questions that we could ask about patients we have known for many years. Do we really know what keeps them bound to us? Are we continuing to engage in a healing process with them? How can we predict whether a life disaster will prove too much for them or for us to bear? What does that even mean? Will it drive us mad? What is madness?

There are, of course, countless questions about our lives and our world that, despite all the efforts of our best thinkers, lack answers. Yet it is just the sort of knowing that cannot be reached by our psychological investigations or even by science or philosophy that seems to call loudly and insistently to us humans. People living in every known society subscribe to some form of religion or spirituality that relies on faith. Some of us are enthralled by magic, some by what may be regarded as pseudoscience—like astrology. According to the American Federation of Astrologers 70 million Americans read their horoscopes daily despite any scientific evidence that they provide meaningful information (Steirwalt, 2020). We would suggest that the answers provided by religion and quasi-religions meet a universal need to reduce the uncertainty of not knowing.

Perhaps this is also why so many of are intrigued by the mystifying province of the uncanny. This strange realm includes the strange coincidences in life that Carl Jung (1952) called "synchronicity." We are reminded of a patient who reported suddenly thinking about a relative and at that very moment received word that he had died. No sooner had a supervisee become aware of an unanalyzed aspect of her traumatic past than she was referred a patient with the very same problem. Are there unconscious aspects of these experiences that have not yet been discovered? Or are unconscious experiences in themselves uncanny?

Freud, who—perhaps more than anyone else—made the world aware of the crucial importance of unconscious experience in psychological life, seems himself to have been fascinated with uncanniness and paranormal phenomena. Both he and Carl Jung were members of the Society for Psychical Research in London. In fact, Freud presented his 1912 paper, "A Note on the Unconscious in Psychoanalysis" to the Society.

Although uncanny experience is not easily explained within his instinctual-drive model, Freud attempted to understand the uncanny in terms of the unconscious processes explicated by his theory. Thus, for example, in his 1919 paper, "the Uncanny," Freud explained: "The uncanny is that class of the frightening which leads back to what is known of old and long familiar" (1919, p. 220). This has become known as "the return of the repressed," or the recalling of what had been lost to unconsciousness.

In his 1919 article, Freud examines many kinds of uncanniness that appear in literature. One story, "Nachstucken," by E.T.A. Hoffman revolves around a gruesome tale of "the Sandman." This fabled character, according to Freud, was "a wicked man who comes when children won't go to bed and throws handfuls of sand in their eyes, so that their eyes jump out of their heads all bleeding. Then he puts the eyes in a sack and carries then off to the half-moon to feed his children" (Freud, 1919, p. 228)

Freud explains the uncanniness in the Sandman story as follows:

> We shall venture, therefore, to refer to the uncanny effect of the Sand-Man to the anxiety belonging to the castration complex of childhood. . . the fear of damaging or losing one's eyes "is often enough a substitute for dread of being castrated".
>
> (Freud, 1919, p. 231)

While we are not convinced that fear of castration is the only way to make sense of the story or even that uncanniness is always experienced as frightening, we find the definition of uncanniness that Freud offers in this article to be highly relevant to our understanding. Explaining how he uses the German word "unheimlich" to capture the meaning of the English word, "uncanny," Freud writes:

> The German word "unheimlich" is obviously the opposite of "heimlich" ["homely"], "heimisch" ["native"]—the opposite of what is familiar; and we are tempted to conclude that what is "uncanny" is frightening precisely because it is not known.
>
> (Freud, 1919, p. 220)

We are struck by Freud's idea that we tend to be frightened by what we do not know—what is unfamiliar, and therefore, more uncertain. We suspect that it is the sense of the unknowable in what we experience as uncanny that leads us to search for explanations that involve the occult or the mystical or even demonic. In other words, uncanny experiences are often accompanied by an intensification of a need to know something for which we have no answers. Perhaps we experience uncanniness when our need to know that there is life after death or that peace, justice and equality are possible, becomes very strong. It may also be that uncanniness is accompanied by an intensification of our need not to know some incontrovertible aspect of reality. We may strongly need not to know that we or a loved one will die, or that we are hurting others or our world. We suspect the need not to know about the traumas associated with World War I greatly affected Freud's account of the uncanny.

John Zilcosky (2018) contends that although Freud never explicitly mentions World War I, there is much in the article that recalls "the return of the fallen and of burial alive in the trenches" throughout the article.

Zilcosky writes:

> The fact that Freud does not connect these traumas directly to "uncanniness" speaks to the problem they pose—for him and for psychoanalytic theory in general. This silence creates an uncanny effect within the essay itself. The Uncanny stages the same "return of the repressed" that it diagnoses. . . The shadow of the war forces us to understand the "uncanny" differently: not just as a personal trauma but as a social symptom of the repression of this suffering.
>
> (Zilcosky, 2018, p. 165)

In agreement with Zilcosky, whom, we believe, admirably identifies implicit references to the horrors of World War I in Freud's article, we also see uncanniness, in part, as reactions to the frighteningly unknowable in world affairs.

We also find it easy to agree with Zilcosky's assertion that the war deeply affected Freud personally. All three of his sons—Martin, Ernst and Oliver—fought in the war and Martin corresponded with him throughout it. What did Freud need not to know that made him omit mention of the war in the article? According to Zilcosky, Freud had often dreamed that his sons had died. In one famous dream, his son, who is out of uniform, his hair gray, had unexpectedly returned home and is hiding in a small storeroom, Freud writes:

> [My son] climbed up on to a basket that was standing beside a cupboard, as though he wanted to put something on the cupboard. I called out to him: no reply. It seemed to me that his face or forehead was bandaged. He was adjusting something in his mouth, pushing something into it. And his hair was flecked with grey. I thought: "Could he be as exhausted as all that?"
>
> (Freud, 1919 [1900], p. 558)

In *The Interpretation of Dreams* (1900) Freud interprets his son's "climbing" as its opposite: his "falling," or dying at war. Zilcosky (2018) notes that Freud failed to see that a troubling aspect of the dream is that his son is not dead but caught uncannily between life and death. Freud's son in the dream bears all the symptoms of war trauma. Freud even states that his son's hair in the dream reminds him of his son-in-law, whose war traumas resulted in his hair turning gray.

Zilcosky advances a dark interpretation of Freud's dream. He writes:

> Not only had he (Freud), like so many fathers, uncritically sent his sons off to war; he had also wished for his son to die, as he admits in the interpretation of his wartime dream, because of "the envy which is felt for the young by those who have grown old." The fact that Freud's dream son is not dead but half-alive and traumatized only increases the guilt. The half-living

> traumatized son, unlike the dead one, never allows the father to complete what Freud calls the "painful" yet
> clean process of leave-taking (Freud, 1919 [1900], p. 560).
> (Zilcosky, 2018, p. 166)

We would say that Freud intensified his need not to know about the fearful dangers the war posed for him and his family. It may even be that, as Zilcosky suggests, he needed not to know about his specific death wishes for his son. We imagine that the intensification of both his need to know and his need not to know fueled his fascination with the uncanny.

We also suspect that Freud's turn away from his original trauma hypotheses played a role in his failure to mention the effects of the war in this article (see Ulman & Brothers,1988; Sletvold, 2016). Sletvold notes that Freud first developed an exclusively trauma-based understanding of the neuroses but then theorized that only sexual trauma and subsequently sexual constitution (sexual-drive-based fantasies and wishes) explains the aetiology of the neuroses (Sletvold, 2016). Sletvold believes that this turn had a very detrimental effect since (childhood) traumas were subsequently neglected for the greater part of the twentieth century by analysts and other clinicians. Brothers (1995) suggested that Freud's unwillingness to acknowledge his own childhood traumas may have contributed to his shift away from a trauma hypothesis.

It is hardly surprising that a catastrophic world event played a role in Freuds' understanding of uncanniness. The writings of complex systems theorists (e.g. Coburn, 2014) help us to understand that the intensifications of the need to know and not to know that emerge in the aftermath of a personal trauma are embedded within complex societal configurations. Consider the premonitions that are often reported on the heels of a societal disaster such as the September 11th 2001 attacks on the World Trade Center in New York. These uncanny experiences seem to play a role in ameliorating both the dread of repetitions of past personal traumas triggered by the disaster as well as the traumatic meanings of the disaster itself. Instead of feeling that one is helpless to combat the horrors that abound in our world, the remembered premonition suggests that something beyond our usual way of knowing is guiding our lives.

We suggest what is experienced as uncanny involves a reversal of the common way that the slippages between what we know on a bodily level and what we need not to know on a cognitive level tend to occur. When something is experienced as uncanny it seems that what we need to know—or need not to know—on a cognitive level does not first involve a body-based experience. It involves an elaboration of something that we have no way of comprehending except by means of imagination or fantasy. An experience of horror or wonder that is body based follows this cognitive knowing.

The Uncanniness of the Doppelganger

Another uncanny phenomenon that Freud extensively discusses in his 1919 article is the experience that one has a double—a doppelganger. This German word, which combines doppel (double) with ganger (goer), refers to a highly uncanny experience of seeing a version of oneself in another person. Doppelgangers appear in such well-known literary works as *Dr. Jeckyll and Mr. Hyde* by Robert Louis Stevenson and *William Wilson* by Edgar Allen Poe.

Freud first refers to the doppelganger in "The Uncanny" by referring to a doll in the Sandman story that seemed to be alive. He suggests that doll-play in some children may be a kind of doppelganger experience. He mentions that the experience of finding a double who looks like oneself is accentuated by mental processes that involve thoughts leaping from one character to the other (he refers to telepathy). This, he suggests, results in the sense of possessing the knowledge, feelings and experience in common with the other.

Freud noted that the uncanniness of the experience is marked by the fact that "the subject identifies himself with someone else, so that he is in doubt as to which his self is." He adds:

> In other words, there is a doubling, dividing and interchanging of the self.
>
> (Freud, 1919, p. 234)

Freud mentions that the double is often associated with "reflections in mirrors, with shadows, with guardian spirits, and with the belief in the soul and with the fear of death." He refers to Otto Rank's idea that belief in the soul as a double was originally "an insurance against the destruction of the ego, an 'energetic denial of the power of death." Rank notes that the "immortal" soul was probably the first "double" of the body.

Freud adds that the invention of doubling serves as a preservation against extinction. He describes his own Doppelganger experience as follows:

> He is in a train's sleeping compartment when the door to the adjoining bathroom flies open and an elderly man in a dressing gown approaches. Assuming that this man is confused and has lost his way, Freud jumps up to set him right, only to realize that the intruder is "nothing but my own reflection in the looking glass on the open door." This shock reminds Freud that he still actually believes that he has a double and, what is more, that he believes this double to be "unheimlich".
>
> (Freud, 1919)

We wonder if the threat of extinction that Freud's doppelganger experience warded off might have been posed by the war or if he was somehow aware that he simultaneous knew and didn't know about the effects of the war on his understanding of the uncanny.

One sort of ominous doppelganger mentioned by Freud is "the evil twin." As Naomi Klein (2023) notes,

> These doubles, who take on our sins so that we can stay pure, are the stuff of monsters in doppelganger books and films: they are the projected selves that get stabbed by the protagonists, who mistakenly kill themselves in the process. These doubles are the unwanted selves that we made some kind of deal with the devil to be free of, now seeking their revenge.
>
> (Klein, 2023, p. 56)

We suspect that many such deals with the devil have been made by people who fall in love and marry others they believe to be their soulmates only to find sometime later that they have married their "evil twin." What did they not want to know about one another when they met? Doris recalls one couple she treated involving an interracial couple. Sarah, who was white was given to outbursts of rage at her black husband, Ed, who seemed incapable of expressing even the mildest form of anger. Interestingly the angry woman was more convinced of her mild-mannered husband's evil nature than her husband was of hers. Sarah was convinced that the passive-aggressive form that Ed's hidden anger took was designed to force her to act out the role of the raging, out-of-control madwoman while he basked in his identity as the calm, gentle, unflappably wise and all-suffering "saint." We suspect that a sort of reversal of the racial stereotypes (black men as aggressive and rageful; white woman as unaggressive and controlled) was probably also at play.

Siblings commonly form such doppelganger matches; one is known as the good obedient child while the other is the troublemaker. We find it important to remember that the evil twin is needed as a repository for the disavowed aspects of the "good" twin. Parents are undoubtedly largely responsible for the creation of child doppelgangers. Their needs not to know about specific aspects of themselves may result in assigning specific characters to their children (see Brothers, 2014, on traumatic attachments).

Doppelgangers in the World

We believe that doppelganger phenomena are pervasive—and often terrifying—in conflicts within personal relationships, within societies and between world powers. Naomi Klein (2023) explicates these conflicts in her 2023 book that is based on her nightmarish experience of being mistaken for Naomi Wolf, a woman whom she believed to hold harmful views that were diametrically opposite the ones she holds dear.

Starting with her own doppelganger experience she references Freud's article on the Uncanny, in which he notes that a person who has a doppelganger may identify himself with another and so become unsure of his true self. Klein observes that "the uncanniness provoked by a Doppelgangers is particularly acute because the thing that becomes unfamiliar (unheimlich) is you" (p. 6).

We would say that the experience of having a doppelganger reflects a particular kind of disturbance in one's need to be known such that the person experienced as one's doppelganger embodies aspects of oneself that are felt to be intolerable.

Klein attributes the stressful, disturbing quality of encountering one's doppelganger to it uncanniness.

Klein sees the images that young (and not so young) people post online as serving as kinds of doppelgangers, mirrors that reflect disavowed aspects of oneself. However, we believe that today's doppelgangers may not always be experienced as disturbing. They may also give expression to wished for aspects of oneself and one's world. Perhaps the images that are so often posted on social media of people in enviably luxurious settings, eating expensive food and of connecting with attractive others reflect this kind of doppelganger. Yet even these pleasant aspects of the doppelganger experience still reflect the absence of some needed way of knowing oneself.

Us-Them and Societal Doppelgangers

For Klein, the doppelganger experience is also reflective of the tumultuous and dangerous times in which we now live. It is not only an individual who can have a sinister double; nations and cultures have them too. Suggesting that she was witnessing, "a new and dangerous political formation," she mentions the "the fascist clown state that is the ever-present twin of liberal Western democracies, perpetually threatening to engulf us in its fires of selective belonging and ferocious despising (p. 12).

In our 2023 book we wrote about fascist experience in terms of the universal tendency to simplify experience in the face of societal traumas as a means of reducing unbearable uncertainty through the creation of the "us vs. them" binary (Brothers & Sletvold, 2023). What we believe is added by viewing societal binaries in terms of doppelganger experience is that it enables us to better understand the need for others to occupy the position of "them." We noted that we tend both to overestimate the similarity of those we consider "us" as well as overestimate the similarity of those we consider "them." The unique individuality of the people included in either group is lost. What is also lost is the sense of ourselves as having all of the human flaws and limitations of those we consider them. Viewing us and them in terms of the doppelganger experience makes it clear that those we deem "them" serve to contain disavowed aspects of those who we include in "us.'

Undoubling

Naomi Klein suggests that a way out of the doppelganger horror is what she regards as "unselfing." It is time, she suggests, "to loosen the grip on various forms of proprietary pain and selfhood and reach toward many different forms of possible connection and kin, toward anyone who shares a desire to confront the forces of annihilation and extermination and their mindsets of purity and perfection (p. 330).

She writes that while, as Freud asserted, confronting one's doppelganger makes one "unfamiliar" to oneself, doing so need not be horrifying. We could not agree more. We believe that not only must we embrace the idea that we cannot know ourselves completely but that we cannot know the other completely either.

We suggest that when we meet one another in the realm of embodied relational knowing it is not unselfing that is needed but rather a humble acknowledgement that, despite our longings, complete knowing, even on a bodily level, eludes us. We are only human.

We end this chapter and our book with a plea that consideration be given to the idea that much in our therapeutic, familial, community and world relationships lies beyond our ability to comprehend. We do not mean to suggest that as analysts we should give up the search for better ways to understand ourselves and others and the world. Rather we hope that by deeply recognizing our limitations, and the strength of our needs not to know and be known, doors to fresh ways of healing and being healed may open before us.

References

Aciman, A (2021). *Homo Irrealis.* New York: Picador, Farrar, Straus & Giroux.

Brothers, D. (1995). *Falling Backwards: An Exploration of Trust and Self-experience.* New York: Norton.

Brothers, D. (2014). Traumatic Attachments: Intergenerational Trauma, Dissociation and the Analytic Relationship. *International Journal of Psychoanalytic Self Psychology*, 9(1): 3–15.

Brothers, D. & Sletvold, J. (2023). *A New Vision of Psychoanalytic Theory, Practice and Supervision: TALKING BODIES.* London and New York: Routledge Taylor & Francis Group.

Coburn, W. (2014). *Psychoanalytic Complexity: Clinical Attitudes for Therapeutic Change.* London & New York: Routledge Taylor & Francis Group.

Freud, S. (1912). A Note on the Unconscious in Psycho-Analysis. *The Standard Edition of the Complete Psychological Works of Sigmund Freud*, 12: 255–266.

Freud, S. (1919). "Das Unheimliche" (The Uncanny). *Standard Edition of the Complete Psychological Works*, vol.17, ed. and trans. by James Strachey (London: The Hogarth Press, 1953), pp. 217–256.

Freud, S. (1919/1900). The Interpretation of Dreams. *The Standard Edition of the Complete Psychological Works of Sigmund Freud,* vols. IV-V. London: Hogarth Press, 1953.

Jung, C. (1952). *Synchronicity: An Acausal Connecting Principle* (1st ed.). Princeton, NJ: Princeton University Press.

Klein, N. (2023). *Doppelganger – A Trip into the Mirror World.* UK/USA: Allen Lane.

Sletvold, J. (2016). Freud's Three Theories of Neurosis: Towards a Contemporary Theory of Trauma and Defence. *Psychoanalytic Dialogues*, 26: 460–475. https://doi.org/10.1080/10481885.1190611.

Steirwalt, S. (2020). Is Astrology Real? *Scientific American.com*, June 25, 2020.

Ulman, R. B. & Brothers, D. (1988). *The Shattered Self – A Psychoanalytic Study of Trauma*. Hillsdale, NJ and London: The Analytic Press.

Zilcosky, J. (2018). 'The Times in Which We Live': Freud's The Uncanny, World War I, and the Trauma of Contagion. *Psychoanalysis and History*, 20: 165–190.

Index

For Product Safety Concerns and Information please contact our EU representative GPSR@taylorandfrancis.com
Taylor & Francis Verlag GmbH, Kaufingerstraße 24, 80331 München, Germany

www.ingramcontent.com/pod-product-compliance
Lightning Source LLC
LaVergne TN
LVHW021506260826
846436LV00056B/389
9781032784380